Hunger, Hope, and Healing

D1016776

HUNGER
HOPE
& HEALING

A Yoga Approach to Reclaiming Your
Relationship to Your Body and Food

Sarahjoy Marsh

SHAMBHALA
Boston & London
2015

Shambhala Publications, Inc.
Horticultural Hall
300 Massachusetts Avenue
Boston, Massachusetts 02115
www.shambhala.com

© 2015 by Sarahjoy Marsh
All rights reserved. No part of this book may be reproduced in any form
or by any means, electronic or mechanical, including photocopying,
recording, or by any information storage and retrieval system,
without permission in writing from the publisher.

Page 219: "Wild Geese" from *Dream Work* by Mary Oliver. Copyright © 1986
by Mary Oliver. Used by permission of Grove/Atlantic, Inc.
Page 271: Excerpt from *Letters to a Young Poet* by Rainer Maria Rilke,
translated by Stephen Mitchell, translation copyright © 1984 by Stephen
Mitchell. Used by permission of Random House, an imprint and division
of Random House LLC. All rights reserved.

9 8 7 6 5 4 3 2 1

FIRST EDITION
Printed in the United States of America

⊗ This edition is printed on acid-free paper that meets the
American National Standards Institute z39.48 Standard.
♻ Shambhala Publications makes every effort to print on recycled paper.
For more information please visit www.shambhala.com.

Distributed in the United States by Penguin Random House LLC
and in Canada by Random House of Canada Ltd

Designed by Steve Dyer

LIBRARY OF CONGRESS CATALOGING-IN-PUBLICATION DATA
Marsh, Sarahjoy.
Hunger, hope, and healing: a yoga approach for reclaiming your relationship
to your body and food / Sarahjoy Marsh.
pages   cm
ISBN 978-1-61180-193-4 (paperback)
1. Eating disorders — Alternative treatment. 2. Yoga — Therapeutic use. I. Title.
RC552.E18M3657 2014
616.85'26062 — dc23
2014014013

This book is dedicated to all those who courageously seek to awaken from and through suffering to love again.

Also to Carmine, Gail, and Jim for your pivotal and loving guidance during periods of suffering in my own life. You provided light, hope, and confidence.

Contents

Acknowledgments

IN THE FALL OF 2010 MY ADMINISTRATIVE assistant, Warren Buss, gave me my phone messages for that day. "Shambhala Publications called to inquire about your work with women. They'd like to know if you would be interested in writing a book." Of course, I'd be honored!

Three years later, I sent the manuscript to Beth Frankl at Shambhala's office. There are numerous people who deserve to be thanked for their support, without which this book would not have come to fruition.

First, the hundreds of courageous women who, since 2001, have attended the workshops, series, and retreats known as "What Are You Hungry For? Yoga and the Psychology of Food and Body Image." These women registered for and attended a course or a weekend without the benefit of having met me through any published readings nor any readily available material on the Internet (which I have been slow to utilize). It is remarkably courageous to sign up for such an intimate and vulnerable event such as a retreat. Many women attended the retreats with no prior yoga experience. Doubly courageous! To those women, many of whom still walk this path together, and to those who have read this manuscript, and offered their hearts along the way, thank you! It is an honor to walk beside you.

Second, adding the undertaking of a book to an already full life cannot occur without the support of persons near and dear:

To my staff at the DAYA Foundation, I would not have been able to turn my attention to this project without your dedication to the yoga therapy programs we provide, the communities we serve, and the partnerships we've created. Thank you to Warren Buss for maintaining just about everything behind the scenes and, especially, for consistently backing up my computer files (something I am too forgetful about myself). To Kate Conwell, who came in just in the nick of time, for taking over the daily operations of studio coordination. Without your support both the book and the community of teachers and practitioners would have suffered. To Lilli Faville, who consistently held the front desk operations together, including walking my little handicapped dog in his wheelchair, and provided me with water, snacks, and assurance every day. To Kerstyn Olson, for your ongoing camaraderie and for always receiving my graphic design delegation so gracefully. To Chelsea Harper, for your groundwork as well as your bird's-eye perspective — and for living a life that is the art of grace and a role model to women everywhere. To Jess Jarris, for your vision and constancy. You see possibilities that have eluded or intimidated me. You make them compelling.

To my students at the yoga studio: thank you for your interest in the material in this book, on behalf of women everywhere. Whether you identified with the issues I have written about or not, your continuous expressions of curiosity, support, and joy were fuel for the writing process.

To the friends who have seen little of me in the last year, and who walked through the ups and downs of life events that occurred while writing this book, I am indebted to you for your patience with me. I look forward to resuming the camaraderie of life as the book moves into the hands of the publishers! A special thank you to Barney McDowell and Judith Roth for reading the first chapter I drafted, "Fervency: Desire and Discipline," and for your enthusiastic responses. You fueled my own fervency and boosted my confidence that this book would work.

And to the most near and dear, my love, Jay Gregory, for your immediate delight about this book project and your ongoing support. As well, thank you for making the meals, tending the garden, building the shed, managing the "small" remodel with much patience, taking on the care and feeding of the household including many pets, and for reading pages of the book while barbecuing dinner. Thank you also for contributing your personal and professional wisdom to my writing process as well as to the content, especially the sections on anxiety, shame, and behavior change. I'm honored to have you as my love, my friend, and my companion. And to the boys, Jason and Ryan, thank you for your patience during school breaks when my "homework" continued and I was unable to "hang out" with you.

For the book's content, I also owe my gratitude to several people, again, without whom the project would not have been completed. To Eden Steinberg for making the first phone call to my studio. To Beth Frankl for picking up the book, guiding me in the early stages of creating a cohesive concept, assigning me an outstanding editor, carrying the manuscript through the stages of Shambhala's acceptance, and, during the most challenging aspects of final submission, for your patience and vision. Thank you for your integrity, heart, and clarity. Karen Levy, your contributions as editor went beyond the words on the page. I am grateful for your clear mind and open heart. You shaped material that is both vulnerable and complex, and brought it to life for those who will be reading it in these pages. You also worked gently with my naïveté along the way, from which my strength as a writer developed. Additionally, Lianne Navedo edited the manuscript for me as part of her yoga therapy internship. Thank you for your attention to detail, your focus, and for bringing your obvious appreciation of the material to all the hours of your editing.

To my photo models, Jess Jarris, Megan Thompson, Keri Olson, Anja Bump, Kate Gray, Julie Gash, and Amarylis Morrow: thank you for offering your practices and bringing joy to the photo shoots. To Alan Weiner: the photographs light up these pages! Thank you for your talent, dedication, and organization. It was a joy to work with you.

As with any undertaking, seeing it through to completion requires certain life skills supported by a sense of our inner compass. In light of this, I also offer my thanks to the core of my yoga and dharma teachers: Catherine Ingram, Jack Kornfield, Shankaranarayana Jois, and Eknath Easwaran. I must also pay homage to the trials and tribulations of my own life—those that imposed learning on me at inconvenient times, those that cleared my heart for the arduous journeys I had yet to begin, and those that created the fires through which I have been transformed. It is to these persons and life teachers that I owe my gratitude.

Introduction

TWENTY-FIVE YEARS AGO I WAS AN ART student in Boston, Massachusetts. At night I was anxious, depressed, lonely, and unsure of myself. I listened to Peter Gabriel's music while the sounds of traffic (both pedestrian and auto) blurred me further into a sense of isolation and being overwhelmed. As he sang "Don't give up . . ." the people and cars outside my apartment had somewhere to go; they had purpose and direction. I did not. I was going down, in a spiral of despair and confusion. During the day, this angst was readily put aside by a sense of purpose I derived from completing art school assignments and monitoring my food intake. Often I failed at the latter, though I exceeded at the former. I relished getting lost in art. Every aspect of my senses felt engaged, and I suspected that art was a medium through which I might be able to save myself. Until nightfall, when I felt despairing again.

This is what it looked like during one season:

The escalation of each new strategy I employed to manage my food intake, to control my body, or to rid myself of the despair brought on by the previous strategy was increasingly accompanied by the escalation of a gnawing disappointment that "this cannot be all there is to life!" I vacillated between exhaustion from and anger at the cycles in which I was caught.

At the time, I did not have the language to describe what was happening to me. I felt certain that what was "happening to me" was only happening to me. I felt incredibly alone, bleak and distressed, usually most painfully at night. Often, this would lift with the arrival of morning and the fresh slate of a new day. A day in which I was going to gain control over myself. A day in which I was going to outrun the behaviors that so powerfully took over my body like an invasion of alien forces. A day in which my normally intelligent, competent, gregarious, and joyful self was going to stay in the driver's seat. And then I would walk by the muffin shop. Only I wasn't able to just walk by — one muffin, and the day was ruined.

I transferred to an art therapy program at a different school. Although it was just across the river from the art institute, my art teachers said they had no knowledge of the practice of art therapy. I sensed I was moving further into the dark, yet with light on the other side.

While I celebrated the world of possibility that art therapy opened up for me, my disordered eating symptoms initially got worse. A significant turning point for me toward recovery occurred neither in art school nor in the art therapy program but on top of a mountain in New Hampshire. Desperate to do something other than downward spiral, I borrowed a backpack from my roommate, rented a car, and drove to a trailhead hours from Boston. I got out, put on my pack, nearly fell over backward from its weight (I overpacked it with things I was going to "do" on my backpacking trip), and began climbing. Hours later I was above tree line and wasted no time taking off my overloaded backpack. As I set it down behind me, I sat on a wide flat rock and lifted my gaze. There before me was 360 degrees of awe. My body, spent from the upward climb with a too-heavy pack, prompted itself to stretch. And I followed. Through the spontaneous movements of my body, years of tension were being released. I experienced an incredible sense of belonging, vastness, unburdened-ness, and ease. The event was so profound that I repeated the stretching exercises every day. When I arrived home to my apartment, I created a mini-routine for myself of fifteen minutes of stretching followed by fifteen minutes of silent sitting each morning. I had a funny-looking purple cushion that I put on the floor to sit on and no yoga gear. In fact, I didn't know what yoga was.

Within a few months of this event, I went to a ten-day silent meditation retreat, and, since the only place to stretch in the mornings was a public exercise room, I discovered that other people were doing similar stretches as my own and that this was called *yoga*.

That was 1989. At that time, I would never have imagined myself having such an opportunity to write to you from a place of complete confidence in life and freedom from all disordered eating patterns and distorted body image issues. My recovery included many of the tools you'll read about here, most notably yoga, meditation, and perseverance. I did not know many of the things you will read in these pages. I did not know what shame was. I did not know what "getting comfortable feeling uncomfortable" was. I did not know what wider circles of empathy were. Yet, as my journey from disordered eating to freedom and authenticity continued, one incremental step at a time, these things were revealed to me in a jolt of immediate understanding. I attribute these immediate understandings to the power of my yoga practice, which made it possible for me to have insight that would become knowledge. Prior to practicing yoga, I'd had countless insights into my behaviors. But insight didn't become understanding; and without understanding, I didn't have new self-knowledge. Without new self-knowledge, I could not have new behaviors.

To give you a glimpse of how I see your recovery, based on my own journey, let me go back to my exhausted, angry, and outraged "this cannot be all there is to life!" self. I didn't want to be caught in the continuous cycles of food chaos, ever circling my shame, fear, body hatred, and self-disgust. Nor was I willing to live a life of weighing and measuring each thing I put into my mouth. Nor did I want to just survive each day white-knuckling my way past all sugar, carbohydrates, or ice cream. I did not want to live each food experience as an exchange to be made up for by certain amounts of exercise to work off the calories. I wanted to live a full-spectrum life where my intelligence, creativity, passion, and genuineness were expressed in my words, actions, friendships, career, and relationships.

My journey started with suffering and, fortunately, was interrupted by awe. From there, I recruited every possible moment and resource to free myself from the suffering that I was imposing. One of the most notable ways that I caused myself suffering was the voice I used to punish, condemn, or "motivate" myself. I started to observe a strong link between the way I spoke to myself and the escalation of symptoms. I noticed an equally strong link between a new way of speaking to myself — with appreciation, forgiveness, and understanding — and my will to keep moving away from self-harm and toward self-nurturance. Incrementally, willingness, self-respect, and faith in myself became my inner motivation.

I have no doubt that the practices of yoga were instrumental in ushering out an old, shaming, unhelpful voice and ushering in a more nurturing, wise, caring voice. Yoga also greatly reduced my anxiety, soothed my exhausted nervous system, and helped me metabolize life events, emotions, thoughts, feelings, and stress. In addition, it became my inner biofeedback machine, letting me know when I was compromising my resilience as well as when I was supporting my mind and heart to move toward love.

I wanted the full-spectrum life I saw from atop that mountain hike. I yearned to experience 360 degrees of possibility as well as permission. My graduate thesis for art therapy centered on this theme and, though that thesis is not the focus of this book, the "360-degree life" is a recovery term I use today in my work with other women finding their way out of suffering and back to awe.

Part One

HUNGER, HOPE, *and* CAPACITY

1

HUNGER

What Are You Hungry For?

Hunger is a deeply primal experience shared across countless life forms and over eons of time. Although all creatures are instinctively wired to satiate hunger, from the smallest lichen-gnawing sea creature to the gazelle-chasing leopard, millions of humans have lost touch with their appetites and their innate intelligence for satiating their hunger. We've also lost touch with the myriad ways in which we experience hunger: hunger for food, for contact, for love, for security, for creativity, for belonging, and so on. As Mother Teresa described, when questioned about why she extended her outreach from the Third World to the West, setting up missions in New York, San Francisco, and elsewhere, "There is hunger for ordinary bread, and there is hunger for love, for kindness, for thoughtfulness; and it is this great poverty that makes people suffer so much."

For some of us, our relationship to our base physical hunger, our appetites, our body, and our very selves has become confused and painful, eliciting feelings of shame, powerlessness, isolation, and despair. Caught in the cycles of bingeing, emotional eating, compulsive eating, yo-yo dieting, or compulsive exercising, we are also caught in the cycles of fear, self-hate, anxiety, depression, hopelessness, and deep doubts about our self-worth. Life becomes a series of strategies to manage these cycles: we feel hopeful about the newest diet or exercise fad we initiate, while also feeling a lurking sense of doom of failing again. I'm writing this book to bring you relief, to support you in stepping out of these cycles.

In the chapters that follow, I'll outline the essential life skills needed to overcome the powerful forces of shame and fear that feed these painful cycles and the self-hate that accompanies them. I'll teach you yoga and mindfulness-based tools for learning these skills in your body, not just in your mind. Throughout the process, you'll learn how to navigate your own journey to complete recovery from these cycles, a recovery that I call "living your 360-degree life."

Hunger and the 360-Degree Life

To begin, we must ask ourselves, "What am I truly hungry for?" We must also ask, "What does 'full' feel like?" "How shall I live 'fully'?" "What does 'empty' feel like?" And "How can I open myself to trusting emptiness?" Addressing the painful relationship to our base physical hunger is a powerful journey from despair, helplessness, and disempowering confusion into our personal strength, resilience, and deep knowing. These are the critical foundations from which we are able to vibrantly address the myriad other hungers that make life worth living and celebrating: the hunger for belonging, presence, creativity, contribution to our community, radiant health, meaningful work, faith, love, and much more. Be assured that the journey you are about to take won't just support you in healing from disordered eating patterns or a distorted body image; it is a journey that will give you the tools and teach you the skills to grow into your 360-degree life. A 360-degree life is much like a balanced relationship to food. It looks like this:

- Hunger and satiation are welcomed experiences: we're not frightened of being hungry; we don't push past satiation to bingeing and numbness.
- Life is full, but not painfully bloated, anxiously busy, or mind-numbing.
- We don't live in cycles of starvation, punishment, mortifying regret, condemnation, or rigid control.
- Life has more flavor, more nuance, and more adventure, all of which we're able to taste and embrace fully.
- We feel, welcome, and know how to respond to our body's urges for rest, exercise, nurturance, and celebration.
- We feel, welcome, and know how to respond to our heart's urges for connection, solitude, soothing, intimacy, inspiration, service, and so on.

the 360-degree life

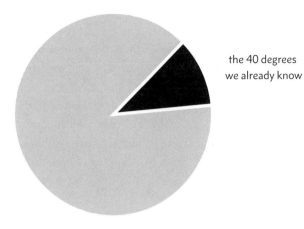

the 40 degrees
we already know

360-degree life
compressed into 40 degrees
by our coping strategies

Figure 1.1

- We're fed by life experiences in the full spectrum: we take in the experience, digest its "nutrients," absorb and integrate what there is to learn, and, following full digestion, become available to what life brings next.

Prior to the journey of recovery, our coping mechanisms compress life down into about 40 degrees of living, rather than 360. If you compress the energy meant to encompass 360 degrees into 40 degrees of space, you will inevitably experience restlessness, frustration, and the urge to break out of that 40 degrees. That is the necessary friction it takes to grow. Currently, you experience that as pain. Soon, you will understand it as fervency.

New Responses to Hunger

Many of us have dull, confused, angry, mushy, or militant relationships to our hungers, both physical and otherwise. We don't know what our body truly craves; we eat out of habit, mindlessly going along with little to no interest in, nor awareness of, what we're truly hungry for.

Or we eat out of the "rule book," which could be what we've read, what we've been told, what we see others doing, or what we decided were the rules of the day, week, or month.

Or we may have a particular craving, but it's long been deemed off-limits. No fried foods, no bread, no carbohydrates, no sugar, no cheese, and so on. Sometimes we have a craving that turns into a binge, reinforcing our belief that our cravings are untrustworthy and bad. But because we may not fully understand our underlying angst toward trigger foods and the power of craving, we repeatedly attempt to maintain control by new means.

Perhaps our relationship to food and hunger is a constant lobbying between deprivation and reward, a mind-occupying negotiation about what we can and can't eat, or a calculated equation of what we have to do to make up for an indulgence.

Perhaps we feel hungry and get annoyed with our body for telling us it needs to be fed. "It's not time yet! It's only 10 A.M., not noon. And besides, you ate the dutiful amount of food for breakfast!" While it is tremendously helpful to examine our hunger to see whether it is a symptom of thirst, anxiety, emotion, or fatigue, it is also helpful to look deeply at the anger we feel toward our appetites when they arise independently of our stated schedule. More often, we address these hungers by trying to tighten the control we have over our biological necessities.

Then there are times when we've eaten past satiation, perhaps even way past, trying to satisfy a hunger of which we aren't even aware, and serving only to make ourselves uncomfortable, or profoundly uncomfortable, and painfully unsatiated in the deepest sense of what it means to be satiated. Often we respond to this with guilt, regret, or shame and with vows to be "better" next time.

As we travel the path of recovery, we have to be willing to be curious, rather than responding habitually or judgmentally toward our relationship to hunger. During my most confused disordered eating periods, I was regularly angry with my body simply because it got hungry. I thought of hunger as a problem, as the enemy, as the damned thing that kept me in trouble with myself, unable to stick to a meal plan or a diet, unable to control my food choices. Having used restricting strategies quite successfully before the binge episodes took over, I was sure that hunger was, in fact, the problem. I did not want to know my hunger. I wanted to annihilate it. But because hunger kept reliably returning, I definitely needed a new relationship to hunger.

To get you started on your 360-degree life, I'm going to ask you to consider three things.

My first consideration would be: What if you were to discover that underlying your currently disorganized relationship to food there is a profoundly intelligent rhythm of hunger and satiation, an intelligent rhythm that has your best interests at heart, an intelligence that can be trusted day in and day out? What if this rhythm is trying to make itself known to you? What if, for every time you keep beating it down by trying to control it, it gets more determined to teach you about hunger and satiation? Perhaps one of the ways it is getting your attention is by making you miserable when you aren't respectful of its innate intelligence!

There are countless critical tasks being done by your body's intelligence all the time. As you read these pages, your lungs are exchanging oxygen and carbon dioxide, your liver is cleansing your blood, your brain is firing synapses, your eyes are taking in letters made into words and meaning, your hair is growing, and your blood pressure is being maintained for homeostasis. All of this is coordinated by your body's intelligence, an intelligence far greater and more intricate than we would ever be able to manage by thinking. That's one of the reasons we don't have to maintain executive function over every part of the body or mind. Imagine how exhausting, daunting, and anxiety producing it would be if we had to manage all of this on our own behalf.

Here is my second consideration for you: What if settling your physical hunger and satiation rhythms into a more intelligent, loving, harmonious relationship freed you to know what your other hungers are? What if underlying your current confusion about your physical hunger is a host of other hungers that you have been literally starving, numbing, or confusing with food? What if there is a similarly primal intelligence that supports your mind and heart to wisely pursue these other hungers?

The challenge is this: we can't know those other hungers while we're overriding and obscuring our ability to respond to our base hunger for food and nourishment. There are other hungers driving you, undoubtedly. They're in there, buried beneath the battles you've been having with yourself. In some ways, we stuff those other hungers down before we even get to know them. In other ways, those hungers are what's rebelling "against" our diet or exercise or self-control plan, causing greater agitation and less relief. Although this is certainly a painful place to be, it is also a tremendous gift because the agitation is forcing you to listen, to take a new approach. You've picked up this book as a part of your new approach. It's time to say thank you to the pain you've been in.

On that note, my third consideration is this: What if this entire mess has been one big symptom, one big blessedly hard symptom that has kept you alive long enough to survive some painful experiences and long enough to get your attention, long enough now to say: it's time. It's time to open up to a new journey. You've been in pain long enough. It's time to take the steps toward your freedom, toward a life you were meant to live all along.

How Hunger Happens

How did we get so hungry? Why is hunger such a restless feeling? How did the other life hungers get there?

The myriad hungers humans experience, such as hunger for companionship, creativity, self-expression, agency, connection, or security, are rooted in one primary hunger: the hunger for love. When we're born, and before we have cognitive abilities, we experience this hunger in a primal, sensory way. We know it when we're bathed in love. We also know it when we aren't. We experience this love when we feel seen, fed, held, contented. Human babies thrive when they are nurtured, lovingly held, properly fed, and attuned to in safe, consistent, supportive environments. Babies twinkle more when we twinkle back at them.

The feeling of being seen, cherished, understood, and cared for strengthens our connection to this primary hunger for love, and satiates it. Alternatively, the feeling of not being seen, not feeling cherished, feeling chronically and painfully misunderstood, or feeling not cared for causes this primary hunger to branch out and make the myriad other hungers unable to satiate us. When we look through this lens, we don't have to keep feeling baffled about why experiences that ought to satiate us don't. When these other hungers aren't or can't be identified, permitted, or soothed, then food (or the control of food) serves to initially satiate, but not for long.

Each human heart longs to be seen. We're born hardwired for this. We're also born vulnerable to the capacity of other humans around us to give us the affirmation that we are cherished for who we are in our uniquely expressed self, and to see us in our humanness. Most of us know the painful experience of feeling unseen, misunderstood, left out, or uncertain about our sense of belonging. If the deep and innate need for belonging weren't hardwired into us, we wouldn't feel flustered when we're misunderstood or when a relationship with one of our special human beings seems threatened. If this deep and innate urge didn't exist in humans, we'd also find a tragically profound deficit in human caring, empathy, and companionship. The innate need to be seen isn't capable, in and of itself, of being a problem. However, when this need goes unmet, how we respond can become problematic, sometimes tragically so.

Here are some compelling things to consider from the teachings of yoga:

1. We're all born as love, as an expression of *ananda*, which translates as love, bliss, or unconditional joy. This ananda is unbroken, unflawed, undiminished, and, at the deepest level, undiminishable.
2. The core of our problems arises from our mind, not our body nor our appetites.
3. Our essence, as love, contentment, radiance, or joy, is unbreakable. Yet an out-of-balance, muddied, or agitated mind can cause us to forget this truth, even to obscure, override, deny, or reject this truth.
4. The journey of recovery is the journey of recovering this deep knowing. It is a journey of homecoming.
5. The deep hunger of the heart to know this truth is one of the core hungers of the spiritual journey. It is a hunger far more powerful and satiable than the ephemeral hungers that many people become lost in or distracted by.

What Else Are You Hungry For?

A 360-degree life has 360-degree hungers. As humans, we have hungers for ease, sanity, faith, direction, creativity, vitality, purpose, connection, hope, harmony, understanding, and countless other deep human desires. Our ability to feel and tend to these hungers gets usurped by food as love, food as reward, or food as punishment. If we are trying to satiate our urge for connection or belonging through food, we'll be hungry underneath. If all we know is how to use food to try to satiate these other hungers, we'll keep trying it with food, even when it's making us unhappy.

On the path of recovery, as you steady your footsteps along the way, you will become aware of the hungers that are deeper than food. When you bring your relationship to food into balance with your body's intelligence, you will be able to feel the other hungers. Through the practices of yoga and self-nurturing discipline, you will also be able to steady your mind and heart when these hungers arise. Even if you don't know how to satisfy the hunger promptly (and often that is why food seems to work so well — it's fairly prompt!), you will feel more confident about your ability to creatively look for solutions. And through the process of recovery, you will feel a deep need to finally satisfy these other hungers that have long been untended, blooming into your 360-degree life: a life of expansiveness and cohesion, a life of possibilities.

2

HOPE
A New Lens through Which to Look

TWO TOEHOLDS

Today, I will claim that I have stepped "two toeholds" [two small
steps one can make even when fear or resistance are activated]
through the door of "recovery." I have been battling this for twenty-
five years and have never felt recovery was truly possible, until now.

—Rebecca, age 40

HOPE

Yesterday, the sun rose over me standing firmly grounded in my
warrior one pose with my arms reaching skyward toward the
heavens . . . I have hope.

—Alice, age 28

A T T H E S T A R T O F A L L O F T H E W O R K S H O P S
and retreats I lead for women struggling with disordered
relationships to food, I say, "There is good cause for hope in this room. You're
all smarter than you feel!" Now, to you, the reader, I say the same thing. You're
smarter than you feel. The choices you have made with addiction were once intelligent, adaptive life skills intended to support your very survival. Everyone's
"life skills" set is generated out of his or her earliest life experiences and experiments. Our early attempts to understand, soothe, enjoy, connect, belong,
or express ourselves, to name a few of our fundamental human needs, were
all mini–research experiments for life. If you've been using food or control of
food, diet, exercise, bingeing, or purging to get understanding, soothing, or

connection, for example, your early research discovered that food, or control of food or body weight (or both), worked to soothe, numb, or distract you, or to create a sense of agency or control, albeit in the absence of actual satiation, soothing, or connection. Food became a medium through which you met your needs. These survival strategies were adaptive and intelligent. Sadly, they then became painfully overused, maladaptive, and ineffective. This leads you to your current circumstance: with a skill set that lacks a diverse set of tools for responding to life.

One of the most problematic pieces of this is also one of the most hopeful: you've outgrown your food, diet, or exercise strategies. (I know you're not completely done using them yet; otherwise, you wouldn't be reading this book.) But your old survival skills aren't working like they did when you were younger. One piece of evidence that you've outgrown these skills is in the frustration you feel that the skills now cause pain. Another is that they no longer work! You may not yet have other, more effective skills for responding to life, so you're in friction with yourself, facing a developmental shift. Just like when you were two years old and faced a development imperative, you may experience frustration, confusion, and clumsiness. Yet I guarantee that if you're reading this book you're outgrowing your old skill set, and you're facing a necessary and exciting developmental shift. Through this process your life is going to be much more amazing than you can perceive it to be from the lens through which you're currently looking.

I know you've already experienced a loss of hope many, many times. "Failed" efforts deflate hope. Hope is the combination of our ability to open up to possibility paired with clear information about our circumstances and a dose of willingness to try something new. I'm here to arm you with clear information about understanding the struggles you've faced and invite you to open yourself back up to hope. With your openness, new skills, and some courage, you can change long-standing behavior patterns. Many students have said to me, "The trouble is, I know what I'm doing isn't good for me. I even know what I should be doing. But I'm not doing it! If I know this, why can't I stop?" The answer is that most of us, at this juncture, have too little information about how our early life decisions became survival strategies and little to no sense of how much we prevent ourselves from being able to move forward by not learning new life skills.

With this in mind, let's pause to appreciate how smart you were. Your young mind came up with a survival strategy that was within your reach, within your power and capacity to execute, even when you were only five, or nine, or fourteen years old. When we acknowledge that a coping mechanism, such as food, works because it provides relief and temporarily soothes (even if soothing is also called comfortably — or uncomfortably — numb), we can understand some of our underlying compulsiveness to keep using food. We know how to put food in our mouths, how to chew, how to hate it while it's happening, how to hit bottom, how to pass out into sleep, how to think "tomorrow will be different," and how to justify and condemn our behavior at the same time. We know how to follow the well-grooved ruts of these behaviors. And we've also come upon a time when this is no longer working. Damning what has been isn't necessary or productive. Damning yourself for doing it also isn't useful. Seeing yourself as facing a friction-filled developmental shift like you had to move through when you were two, and seven, and twelve, and sixteen may help you feel more hopeful. It's also likely that some of the work you were meant to do during biologically driven, psychosocial developmental shifts didn't happen fully. In a case like that, we may experience the shift only partially, leaving us reliant on the survival strategies that we knew how to manifest at that time. On the one hand, this is merciful by design: we didn't have the environment (people, support, social circumstances) to navigate these developmental shifts and help us generate new skills, and we weren't stripped of the ones we were able to develop. Also, mercifully, what we weren't able to do then, we have the opportunity to do now.

If we can approach the processes of change from the perspective of appreciation for the brilliance of our early choices, we'll be able to move forward with kindness, perspective, and hope, rather than overwhelming ourselves with self-hatred, condemnation, and the alternating feelings of chaos and rigidity that accompany the cycles of painful behaviors (which become compulsions and addictions). The tools of yoga, as well as the embodied practices, teach us the skills to make these changes — and not just in our minds but rather down to our bones, into our vitality, into our deep and wise knowing. This is worth mustering the hope for!

It's time for me to arm you with information about the roots of your current behaviors so as to disarm your ability to think you just haven't been smart enough. Truly, in your early efforts to survive, you were smarter than you feel today. And the pain you're in now is good cause for hope — because you aren't willing to settle for living the way you have been. In the spirit of clear information, let's look more closely at how disordered eating patterns have been a survival skill.

- To survive distress, dis-ease, and discomfort, to bear painful experiences, confusion, fear, and pain, you needed to create a survival skill. Because substances take away pain, food (emotional eating, binge eating, and attempts to control food through dieting, restriction, or elaborate plans) became a tool you used to survive. It was a skillful adaptation at the time you turned to it. It was a once-adaptive effort to gain some control over the feelings of discomfort that you didn't know how to manage, explore, or understand.
- If you didn't have support, loving mentoring, or permission for your discomfort, you didn't internalize the life skill of identifying discomfort as a normal human occurrence, as a signal that something is awry, or as a sign that you're experiencing a growth opportunity.
- If you were blamed for other people's distress or subject to the whirlwind of other people's compulsive activity, chaos, or rage in the face of distress, you likely learned that discomfort is bad, that it can cause harm to self and others, that you are a source of discomfort to important people (such as parents), and that discomfort should be avoided in all possible ways.
- With such deep learning at a time when your brain was developing its foundation — its operating system, to use a computer analogy — your discomfort-management strategies, which have become disordered eating patterns, were essentially deeply programmed into you. The obvious manifestation of compulsive or disordered behaviors may not arise until a later point in life when more subtle or acceptable discomfort-management strategies stop working. This might show up when your stress levels escalate and your discomfort increases, as in losing someone close to you, leaving home for college, getting married or divorced, losing a job, and so on.

Why does it keep happening? Here are some main reasons.

- Addiction, once begun, basically programs you to run its course again and again.
- Addiction successfully repeats the same outcomes again and again.
- Even if those outcomes are painful and confusing, they're also familiar. To our addiction-programmed, discomfort-avoidance patterns, familiar pain is better than unfamiliar pain.
- When distress arises, addiction is programmed to pop up first on the options screen.
- We've honed these behaviors into finely tuned life skills, strategies to manage pain.

～≈ I use the terms *disordered eating patterns* and *addiction* to refer to the various ways in which symptoms may present. I define *addiction* to mean the cyclical or repetitive reliance on behaviors and coping mechanisms (usually painful) to self-medicate, avoid, or manipulate our experiences (feelings, moods, body events, stress, joys, sorrows, and so forth). Addictive behaviors and coping mechanisms create life symptoms: they prevent us from living with honesty and integrity with ourselves or others, cause harm to ourselves or others, diminish our self-respect, or create poor health or dis-ease (physical or mental). Addiction may be to a substance, an activity, or a relationship. In this regard, addiction is not a "bad" thing. It is a behavior cycle.

We all need skills to survive. Primitive people used skills that we no longer need today. The skills we have now, like central heating, would have been completely impossible for them. All species evolve and adapt to their environment, usually quite slowly. So, too, can you. You can develop new and healthier survival skills, and you can develop the skills and tools you'll want and need to thrive. (I'd like to see you do more than survive. I'd like to see you thrive!) This book teaches you the skills you need to get started on your recovery and offers you the tools to stick with it.

THE CYCLE OF ADDICTION

It started as a plan for what I would eat and when. I felt confident, elated, and in control. Life was manageable, and I was going somewhere! The scale proved it. My clothes showed it, too.

The plan got more creative, and more severe. It was easy to follow — most of the time. Riding my bike or walking long distances made up for the times when I couldn't follow the rules (of the plan). I felt in control — most of the time. Berating myself made up for the times when I couldn't follow the rules.

I broke the rules much more often. I did not feel I was in control. I wondered how I'd lost so much control and made efforts to get it back. I read, researched, and dreamed up ideas of my own [to manage the "out-of-control" side and to stay in line with the "in-control" side].

The battle got more severe. My out-of-control side threatened, lurked, taunted me to eat this, eat that, just one more bite, just one more time, just this last ice cream cone, the last one ever. Don't worry about it. You'll make up for it tomorrow. Walking, biking, food restriction routines . . . you can make up for this tomorrow.

Down the rabbit hole with Alice . . .

I would wake up from time to time and wonder, "How did this get to have so much control over me when I was trying to have control over it?! How did I lose control, when I'd had it so good before?"

The cycle of addiction has common rhythms to it, though its shape may change slightly or be nuanced in one area or another for each of us individually. At times, the shape of my cycle described above was more oblong, moving rapidly from the "Plan" to the "Episode." At other times, I'd craft a plan that actually seemed to work for a while, keeping me under control. Until it didn't; until I'd "slip" . . .

Sometimes this entire cycle starts with what our culture would think of as an innocent urge to go on a diet, lose some weight. Yet the diet industry is out of tune with hunger, appetite, satiation, and the nature of individual nutritional needs. As such, 95 percent of diets set people up to fail. Then, because the *diet fails . . . they fail . . . reinforcing* feelings of failure around food, weight, and getting "control" over the body and all of its "messy" needs and feelings. There is a fundamental thing to know about the impact of a diet on your brain function: you can set yourself up for very disordered thinking and metabolic functioning by going on a diet without proper medical and nutritional guidance. Some of the diets people put themselves on are literally starving their brain of essential nourishment. This will change brain function, cause biological cravings (your brain asking for something from your body), cause your body to work harder to maintain homeostasis, set you up for bingeing, and shift your metabolism, making it harder to lose weight even when you eat healthfully. Fortunately, with recovery and proper care and nutrition, you can revive this functioning. I include this perspective here because I hope it will free you from blaming yourself if specific diets have failed and you're telling yourself you just don't have enough willpower, or if this cycle started for you with an "innocent" diet and then you no longer recognized your own thinking.

the cycle of addiction

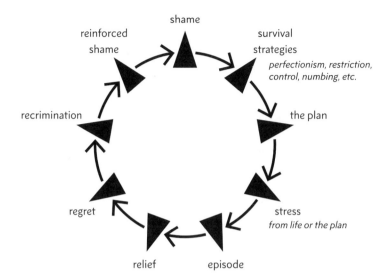

Figure 2.1

What I'm outlining in the cycle of addiction is the result of decades of recovery, years of working with women through these processes, and continued professional study. As you read, perhaps you'll identify with aspects of this cycle, or perhaps you'll see yourself entirely in this cycle.

Shame

At the core of all addictive processes is the base experience of *shame*. Whether the addiction is to a substance (such as food, alcohol, or cigarettes) or behavior (for instance, gambling, work, or sex), the compulsive urges to numb, protect, harm, or deny our selves are rooted in the core sense of shame. With a foundation of shame at the core of our being, we'll be prone to struggling with feelings such as anxiety, fear, depression, a sense of being overwhelmed, and urges for control, security, and safety.

Survival Strategies

To help manage the painful experience of shame, we create *survival strategies*, finding ways to escape, numb, purge, hurt, or damn ourselves. And, paradoxically, this truly feels like relief. Food provides a tremendous relief to the swirling sensations of emotions we may not even register moving through us. Purging brings on relief, including the physiological rush. Restricting food also has a biochemical effect on our body, mind, and heart. While these varieties of relief are generated by seemingly opposing behaviors, each of these processes empowers us to have a direct and dramatic impact on our body and mind. The fact that we can do it to ourselves is critically important to understand. These behaviors started as attempts to survive, find safety, and have some control over what was happening within us, even when that was stimulated by what was happening around us.

Quite often, we're very young when these processes are getting formed, so our brain is not yet capable of more complex thinking or problem-solving. When we reach for substances to manage pain, that's relatively primitive (reflecting a very early stage of development). What we can turn to for relief would have to suit the developmental stage of our brain—and at early ages, this would include things that we can eat, ingest, or do to our physical body. It would include things like overeating or restricting foods, drinking, dieting, purging, or controlling (or trying to control) physical urges like hunger, elimination, or even rambunctiousness.

One of the critical things to understand is that we generated these tactics because we could. We had what it took to reach for food. We had what it took to purge, to starve, to self-harm. We were terrified, overwhelmed, confused, or sad; and we had no idea how to feel such things. Nor did we have the support in place to help us.

So we started using these tactics to spare ourselves further terror, pain, or confusion. The more we turned to these behaviors, the more deeply fixed and subconscious the choices became—until there was no longer a choice; "it" had taken control of us. What started as an understandable and relief-inducing strategy became an overwhelming and painful cycle.

The Plan

We created strategies that became deeply grooved behaviors. Today, when those behaviors get out of control, we make a *plan* to get them back into control, whether that is how we will get through this day, this meal, or this week. Usually, the plan involves arrangements about which foods we can eat, how much we can eat, how we will exercise, how much weight we need to lose to become acceptable again, how we will get ourselves back under control, and so on. The plan is the mental process, the tangible representation of our attempts to overcome shame. The plan is generated without reference to, or respect for, our body's actual needs, capacities, and hungers.

This plan is our attempt to feel better, to make ourselves more acceptable to those around us, and to capture the feelings of love and security that seem so elusive. In our minds, at the time we make the plan, it seems perfectly reasonable that if we ate only eight hundred calories in a day, then we would be deemed worthy of going on. Or that if we managed to eat only apples for the day, and we managed to be successful at that, then that would be a measure of our worth and competency. Very often the plan is laced with ideas about how to make ourselves perfect, acceptable, and worthy of inclusion in family or community or culture, and to get a grip on feelings of loss of control, chaos, confusion, and pain.

When the plan is working, we experience buoyancy, elation, and feelings of competence and safety. We've employed a variety of ways to be in control, temporarily, of bodily functions, but also of thoughts, emotions, and needs. However, if we learned that our bodily functions, emotions, or needs were messy, burdensome, wrong, bad, or intolerable to others, then we may struggle more to allow ourselves to live in the base intelligence and the ever-changing nature of our body.

Stress

The plan is put in place to prevent distress or a host of other feelings, all of which are much more difficult to be with when our root shame goes unnoticed. Because the plan is not usually crafted with tender and encouraging respect for the body, it will be unachievable, undoable. Eventually, the *stress* of the plan builds. Paired with life's stressors, we're setting ourselves up to fail. Because we have been using food or related behaviors as a coping mechanism, our capacity to handle stress with alternative skills is seriously underdeveloped.

The Episode

When stress hits its high point, we reach for our long-repeated behaviors to manage it. Just as a thousand times before, our longtime coping mechanism works! Whether it's two bites of a brownie, three extra raisins, or an all-out binge-purge. Whatever the choice in our addiction, behaviors, rituals, I call this part of the cycle the *episode*. We binge; we have an episode. We purge; that's an episode. We eat manically in the car; that's an episode. We shove three cookies in our mouth hurriedly; that's an episode.

Relief

Initially, and almost instantly, this brings on feelings of *relief* from the stress. The body registers a biochemical infusion of relief. For a few moments, minutes, or sometimes hours, we feel numb to what was causing the stress. We get to feel numb, and that mercifully numbs us to the underlying but unnamable feeling of shame.

Regret

This is followed immediately by (or co-arising with) great feelings of *regret*, profound disappointment, frustration, self-recrimination, anger, and implosion. Even when we're reaching for the brownie or the three cookies, competing voices may be screaming their familiar taunts—"You'll never get over this! See how weak you are? You couldn't even last one day!"—or championing their causes—"Just this one and then we'll start over. Things just got too intense this one time; don't worry about it. Okay, one last time through the drive-thru. Then we'll stop!" With enough repetition of this cycle, we already know the profound regret waiting for us after the episode.

Recrimination and Reinforced Shame

In the flush of this, we fall into feelings of *recrimination and reinforced shame*. We become punitive, angry, and self-condemning. In this way, our long-ago internalized feelings of shame are reinforced. We've just behaved in ways that mightily reinforce our shame, our badness, our incompetence, our worthlessness. And we are very unkind with ourselves in these moments. This part of the cycle is when we reinforce the original messages and feelings of deep shame. We know we're worth berating and condemning. We just proved how hopeless we are, after all!

The Plan

Having no other route out and not knowing what to do with the mess we just made, we rally ourselves to reconcile this terrible shame with another plan (or the same plan) to start the next day, the next week, or the first of the month. Often, it becomes more punishing and unrealistic as the cycle continues. We feed the cycle (pun intended!) every time we plan unrealistically, plan from self-hatred, plan to grasp at control, or plan without other coping mechanisms in place. And yet, when we are making plans from the recrimination and shame stage, we can't help but make plans that become a part of the self-sabotaging, shame-reinforcing cycle of addiction.

Finding Your Way Out

Very often when I discuss the cycle of addiction with the women in my groups, a quiet stunned look comes over their faces. They instantly identify with the cycle. They see themselves in it, and the long-held belief that they were the *only* ones who experienced this "craziness" is suddenly over. "That describes me!" they'll exclaim. "I thought I was the only one doing this weird stuff." "How did you know what I was thinking?" One of the most painful things about a food-centered addiction or body-centered self-hatred is the utter feeling of aloneness in it all. With these behaviors, secrecy and isolation are ubiquitous. Thus, the feeling of revelation that comes over women in my groups when they see this cycle illustrated and discover that it intimately describes their thinking process is tremendous cause for hope: they are not and have not been alone, and they are not just doomed to repeated failure.

This reduction in the sense of isolation is one of the powerful tugboats that can pull us out of being stuck in the cycle. Ultimately, finding our way out involves the following:

- New coping skills that you can embody.
- The conviction that you can step out of the cycle anywhere along the spectrum, including the interruption of a binge. In other words, you don't have to wait to hit "bottom" in your cycle in order to interrupt it. In fact, that thinking is a part of the cycle — which I recommend you strongly resist.
- A clear enough self-will not to punish yourself with more severe plans.
- A clear enough mind not to initiate an unrealistic plan. (And a clear enough mind to initiate a realistic plan.)
- Self-awareness and sensitivity skills to feel stress or other body-mind experiences before they become triggers, and a willingness to learn how to relate to and respond to these experiences differently.

- New skills—did I say that already?! If this is going to be more than just a dreamy idea, then we *must* learn new skills for coping with life's messy uncertainties. These life skills must be skills we can do with our mind and body, and they must address the physiological experiences of anxiety, confusion, excitement, hope, and feeling overwhelmed.

Yoga is an ideal vehicle for this learning.

Why Yoga Is Different from the Other Things You've Tried

If you're pursuing recovery the way that I did, then you've tried many things already. What I have found through my personal experience, and now through two decades of professional experience, is that recovery strategies that only treat the symptoms won't work. Yoga teaches us that symptoms are reflections of underlying issues in the mind. Our symptoms are trying to get our attention to steer us toward a deeper journey. We're not meant to live a life of symptom-management strategies. Managing our symptoms won't lead us to the gem hidden within our symptoms; our symptoms tell us that we have unmet needs (for stability or safety, for example), deeper desires (for creativity and sensuality, for example), and hidden anxieties that are urging us to grow. Yoga is a body-centered approach to recovery, and it recognizes that all symptoms arise with a body-and-mind component. Yoga addresses the underlying fear that keeps symptoms in play, integrates recovery tools that are body- and mind-centered, and has documented success in recovery.

Yoga Addresses the Underlying Fear

Symptoms that become out of control (like disordered eating patterns) generate an undercurrent of anxiety and fear. This fear narrows our attention to whatever seems to be the threat and focuses our attention on our symptoms, because they are obvious. However, our symptoms aren't actually the threat; they are simply telling us that we feel threatened on some level and we don't know how to navigate it.

Additionally, a hurdle many face is the fear of recovery. Students tell me they are afraid of living without their familiar coping mechanism, or frightened of what life will be like when they are healthy. They become afraid of failing again, or frightened of how the choices they will have to make for recovery will upset others. These fears are normal. If you've been out of control lately, then fear can arise in the process of reining yourself back into your body. If you've become accustomed to feeling in control via more and more rigid strategies, then opening up your 360-degree life is going to feel frightening.

Because people are generally afraid of the unknown (yes, people all over are afraid of the unknown), the unknown, if it continues to be scary, will prevent us from recovering. Without a tool kit that is embodied — rooted in the body — to help us negotiate this fear, we will continue to face setbacks on our path to recovery.

Fear ignites our fight-flight-freeze-submit circuitry. *Fight* demands our aggression toward a perceived threat, much like a dog barking or attacking. *Flight* tells us to run or escape, much like a cat fleeing a loud noise. *Freeze* immobilizes our decision making as we scan the enemy or threatening territory looking for ways out, like a deer caught in the headlights of a car. And *submit* mimics resignation or death, much like the possum. (You may be familiar with this process as the fight-or-flight response. My initial training in mental health included fight or flight as the two responses that our reptilian brain uses under threat. In recent years, research has expanded our understanding of this to include the freeze and submit responses as well.) Yoga quiets the anxieties of the mind and allows the biochemistry of love, hope, and self-respect to enter. Yoga helps us shift from fear to opportunity, from confusion to patience, and from chaos to clarity.

YOGA MOMENT

Stretching to Dissolve Fear

Unresolved fear or anxiety continues to circulate in our body-mind system. Communication between body and mind is an intimate reciprocity. What remains unresolved in body will influence the mind; what remains active under our conscious mind will affect the body as each seeks resolution. Yoga dissolves the held patterns of unresolved fear (as well as unresolved frustrations, disappointments, and so on) bit by bit. You'll read more about this in the chapters to come. For the moment, try this:

- Seated or standing, interlace your fingers.
- Then turn your hands inside out and stretch your arms up overhead.
- Squeeze your arms to straighten the elbows and actively stretch your entire spine.
- Breathe deeply through your nose and into your belly five times.
- Release your arms and observe your body's response to the stretching and breathing. You may have the urge to yawn or move the upper back, neck, or shoulders. You might feel a tiny bit more vibrant or relaxed.

When we stretch muscles and breathe properly, it alerts our body's system to remove stress, tension, and the biochemical waste products of each. Bit by bit, we dissolve stored fears, sadnesses, frustrations, and other feelings, too.

Yoga Integrates All Aspects of Recovery

Yoga is an integrated, holistic, 360-degree approach to life, addressing all aspects of recovery. Even if we used yoga just to manage the fear we face about behavior change, because yoga addresses our entire being, it will eventually deeply penetrate, in a kind and gentle manner, our mind, which will transform how we relate to our body, psyche, heart, breath, and consciousness.

Yoga also integrates the left and right hemispheres of the brain. As yoga and mindfulness tools slow down the mind and balance the hemispheres of the brain, we begin to experience (1) a sense of relief from the cycles of self-harm and self-criticism and (2) an ability to access spacious self-understanding and forgiveness. From this, transformation occurs. (No one ever got better by damning themselves out of their addiction, or shaming themselves out of their inner critic!) Because yoga is a body-mind activity, we have the opportunity to open up to our right hemisphere's gifts: timelessness, spaciousness, contentment, loving-kindness, and equanimity. If you've only tried to recover through linear, logic-based strategies such as thinking of new schemas, planning new diets, evaluating your progress with militant standards, criticizing your downfalls while hoping to motivate yourself to stop unhealthy behavior, or creating logical, rational, even mathematical equations as to how to spend your time, eat proper meals, or schedule your day to avoid compulsive behaviors, an approach that incorporates yoga will be a breath of fresh air (pun intended). A whole new world will open up as you include your body, heart, and intuition

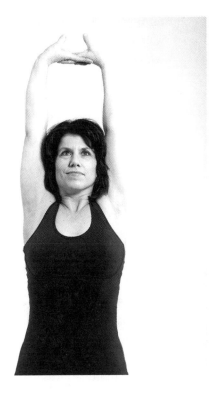

in your recovery process. This will awaken your hope and build your capacity for wise living.

Yoga Has Documented Success

Another good cause for hope at this juncture of your recovery: the demonstrated success in using the practices of yoga to overcome addiction of all kinds. In a recent search for eating disorder treatment centers that include a yoga program in their treatment plan, I reviewed twenty centers in America. In this review, 80 percent of these residential treatment centers offer yoga classes as part of their exercise program and 30 percent offer yoga therapy programs (individual yoga therapy sessions with a trained yoga therapist).

Yoga has helped many women with disordered eating patterns learn to accept their body and recover from their behaviors. A study published in *Psychology of Women Quarterly* (June 2005) reported that mind-body exercises such as yoga are associated with greater body satisfaction and fewer symptoms of disordered eating than traditional aerobic exercise such as running or using cardio machines. Cardio workouts tend to be driven by calorie-burning or weight (or shape) management. Yoga suggests motivations of self-acceptance, self-awareness, and relaxation.

Yoga and meditation reduce negative body-image thoughts and emotions, provide relaxation of the mind and body, create positive body awareness, and reduce stress. Those of us who have been using food to manage stress and emotions have learned to suppress and ignore the natural sensations of our feelings and our body. Yoga encourages a new and very hopeful exploration of natural sensation, feelings, desires, body signals, and mental habits.

Yoga Is for Recovery and for Life

What, exactly, is yoga? It is a series of physical exercises done to invigorate, cleanse, detoxify, and restore the body. It is breathing practices done to soothe anxiety, overcome fatigue, and balance the hemispheres of the brain. It is the art of concentration. It is consistent, deliberate effort toward stilling the mind. It is a state of being, a state of realization in which we rest unself-consciously in luminous, open, receptive awareness. It is a philosophy of life. It is nothing short of a pathway addressing our mind-body-heart-spirit, a pathway that teaches us to live in harmony with ourselves, with each other, and with life itself.

The practice of yoga might start with the physical body, the palpable, tangible body of muscles and bones. Yet its impact cannot be contained to the muscles and bones. When we stretch the muscles, we're opening our muscles to new ways of holding ourselves in the world. Simultaneously, we're opening our muscles to fresh circulation, which means a better delivery and transport system for all of the nutrients, chemical messengers, and necessary nourishment for the body as well as the removal of waste products being held by tension patterns. Yoga teaches us how to relate to and respect our vitality.

Yoga also stretches us into feeling, intuition, and a connection to the source of our hungers, both mundane (like craving broccoli, rice, or bananas) and spiritual (like craving purpose, creativity, or liberation). Through the process of releasing layers of physical tension, mental or emotional disconnection, fatigue, or numbness, we discover our long-forgotten selves, and our resilience, grace, and ease. We become able to welcome and respond to the deepest hungers of our body, heart, and spirit with fresh awareness and greater skillfulness.

Yoga's perspective on recovery addresses our whole selves:

- Yoga sees behaviors as results of deeper processes. Behaviors are symptoms of underlying experience, messengers that we're out of balance with ourselves.
- Yoga addresses brain chemistry by increasing circulation and respiration.
- Yoga quiets the nervous system, de-fogs depression, and soothes anxiety.
- Yoga improves digestion, endocrine, and immune function by shifting us from the adrenal response to the relaxation response.
- Yoga shifts us from the sympathetic to the parasympathetic nervous system.

How does all of this help with recovery? Yoga provides tools for coping with the trials and tribulations of letting go of addictive patterns. We learn skills through the practice of the yoga poses. We learn to allow for feelings and sensations that might otherwise be uncomfortable, feelings that we might otherwise want to escape. Here are some ways yoga does this:

- Yoga teaches us to become present to ourselves.
- Yoga teaches us to notice the restlessness of the mind and our urge for escape hatches.
- Yoga gives us a place to focus the mind, learn to concentrate, and become aware of our mental habits.
- Yoga teaches us the process of learning to listen deeply, respond wisely, and care lovingly for our body, mind, and heart.
- Yoga is a 360-degree approach to living with vitality, ease, presence, intuition, confidence, and self-acceptance.
- Yoga teaches us to experience emptiness and fullness from a new perspective.
- Yoga breaks us out of the spell of isolation — and shame — as we realize our struggles are the struggles of humans everywhere.
- Yoga teaches us how to cultivate greater self-intimacy and acceptance.
- Yoga teaches us how to trust the larger pulse of life.

What yoga is *not*:

- It is not another control technique.
- It is not another perfectionism project.
- It is not another food-management strategy.

- It is not another black-and-white-thinking device. ("I took my yoga class, I deserve a brownie." "I didn't go to yoga, I'm no good.")
- It is not another self-condemnation device.
- It is not a process of ruthless self-examination or criticism.
- It is not another place to induce shame or hide out from feelings.

Still, when it comes to food and related issues with disordered eating, how can yoga become a realistic alternative? At the start of my workshops, I've asked hundreds of women the question "How has food helped?" Later, at the end of the workshop I've asked, "How does yoga help?" The similarities are remarkable:

HOW HAS FOOD HELPED?	HOW DOES YOGA HELP?
Creates connection (through food)	Creates connection (with ourselves)
Soothes	Soothes
Ignites belonging (family, comfort foods)	Ignites belonging (to a community of other practitioners)
Creates a time-out	Creates a time-out (from stress)
Provides a treat / reward	Provides a treat / reward
Expresses rebellion	Provides a rebellion against _____
Softens the sorrows	Softens the sorrows
Puts us in a trance (numb)	Puts us in a trance (meditative)
Shifts energy / biochemistry	Shifts energy / biochemistry
Awakens creativity (cooking, food combining, meal planning)	Awakens creativity (spontaneity, curiosity)
Increases love (whether we feed ourselves or others)	Increases love (deep self-care + self-respect)
Provides pleasure	Provides pleasure
Creates illicit pleasure	Transforms illicit pleasure into healthy indulgence
Creates secrecy (personal secret others don't know)	Transforms secrecy into prioritizing personal worth
Numbs the pain	Numbs the pain
Makes the unbearable more bearable	Makes the unbearable more bearable
Helps with anger management	Helps with anger management

| Provides personal time (savoring something just for us) | Provides personal time (renewing, restorative) |

We've been using food to meet specific needs. Valid needs. Yoga creates a more skillful and viable option for meeting those needs, without the mental and physical side effects of food strategies.

HOW IS THIS GOING TO WORK? YOGA'S TRIPOD FOR RECOVERY

As we venture forth into the body, mind, and heart of this work, I'd like to give you a sense of how I map the recovery terrain. Yoga has a system called *kriya yoga* that acts like a tripod for your recovery. It's the tripod of discipline, self-study, and surrender, also known in Sanskrit, the language of yoga, as *tapas, svadhyaya,* and *isvari-pranidhana.*

Sadly, many of us have engaged these three tools detrimentally. Unhealthfully, tapas becomes rigid control strategies prepared to punish; svadhyaya becomes painful self-examination or endless cycles of asking "Why am I

the tripod of yoga

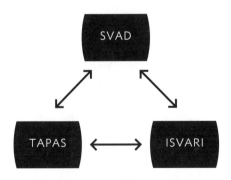

UNHEALTHFUL

tapas: rigid control strategies, punishment
svadhyaya: painful self-examination,
endless cycles of "why am I doing this?"
isvari-pranidhana: resignation, apathy, giving up

Figure 2.2

the stages of recovery

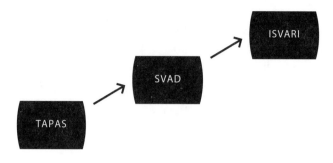

HEALTHFUL

tapas: self-nurturing discipline

svadhyaya: self-study and self-empathy

Figure 2.3 isvari-pranidhana: forgiveness and freedom

doing this?" without resolution; and isvari-pranidhana becomes resignation or apathy.

Rather than using a strict tripod model, it's been my experience that using a stages-of-recovery model better prepares you for your full recovery, your 360-degree recovery. Discipline (tapas) becomes the foundation. With discipline as the foundation, we essentially place ourselves at the trailhead of an amazing journey. The terrain of recovery is sometimes bumpy, sometimes easeful, sometimes steep, and sometimes profoundly scenic and joyful in unexpected ways. A step-by-step process builds a reliable, lifelong foundation for recovery that then healthfully incorporates self-study and surrender. Based on my years of experience with both recovery and yoga, I have found this linear process helpful with the nonlinear process of the journey.

Fervency/Discipline: We begin with fervent discipline, tapas, to commit to a path of sobriety and place deliberate focus on self-nurturance to create incremental change toward the goals of health and freedom. Through yoga and personal commitment, we cultivate self-nurturing discipline, learn new life skills, and apply those life skills daily to internalize them as our go-to responses to life.

Self-Study and Self-Empathy: Once we establish a measure of sobriety, we'll have more skills and more confidence in the process (and in ourselves). Then we go more deeply into self-study, svadhyaya, into understanding the underlying material that's been feeding our issues all this time. In this process, we rediscover faith and courage, develop greater self-empathy and attunement, become more respectful of our resilience, and develop our strength in countering self-abandonment. We know we will not give up on ourselves.

Forgiveness and Freedom: At this stage, we learn self-forgiveness at its best. With deep self-understanding, empathy, and respect, we practice radical self-forgiveness. We see ourselves through an entirely different lens than we've known before: the perspective of love, wisdom, and belonging. Through surrender, isvari-pranidhana, we become capable of "widening our bandwidth" in life beyond painful coping mechanisms to freedom from self-harming, self-demeaning, and self-diminishment. We become free of such urges and the misunderstanding that drove those urges early on. When it comes to this stage, surrender won't be as terrifying as it might seem now.

In the following chapters of this book, I'll be offering you tools, yoga exercises, and skills for building your recovery. It's likely that you will have times of confidence, excitement, and relief. Yet you may also have times where you feel overwhelmed, frightened, or resistant. I strongly recommend that you move through the chapters in stages and adopt the suggestions along the way. As you integrate one new skill, it will be the foundation for other skills to sprout into strengths.

Why Discipline First?

Let's think about this in terms of the trailhead metaphor. In order to get ourselves to the trailhead, we have to take action. We have to deliberately place ourselves in the momentum of arriving at the trailhead. Thinking *about* the trailhead is not the same as being *at* the trailhead. Planning elaborate ideas about how to get to the trailhead or reading about trailheads won't do it either. I know the urges for each of these. During my own recovery, I did a lot of thinking, planning, reading, and "preparing myself to be prepared" to get started, take action, or get restarted.

The question of why we focus on discipline first deserves a larger and more hopeful answer. Some of the most significant reasons we don't get started more easily in recovery include the following:

1. I don't know how to do it.
2. I won't know how to do it.
3. I won't know what to do when I get lost.

4. It is too scary.
5. It will be too scary.
6. I have been doing this [behavior] for too long.
7. I won't know what else to do when I am stressed.
8. I will have to feel things that I don't want or know how to feel.

No one knows how to do something new and courageous before they do it. The part about recovery being scary feels very, very real. I know. But with the teachings in this book about discipline and self-care, and about other supports you can create in your life, you will know what to do when you get lost or when you feel overwhelmed or scared. For the work I do with women, I use the word *fervency* to reflect the quality of discipline we will need to recruit for recovery: at times it will be fiery, at times fierce, yet always focused toward the goal of re-covery. (Discipline, in this sense, is never used to punish.) You will read about this in chapter 4.

The hopeful news about using fervency, or discipline, first in recovery is that as you start hiking, you will only be required to put one foot in front of the other. You will only be required to stay on course in small increments.

Many women have told me that in order to move toward recovery, they will first have to sort out years of stored feelings. Thinking that you have to sort out your feelings before you can start the journey of recovery is one of the major postponements to recovery. And, it's an illusion. Many feelings are repeated feelings, self-stirred feelings from the cycles of addiction. We actually can't know the feelings underneath our behaviors while we're still actively engaging in those behaviors. We can only feel how painful our behaviors are. This can be profoundly deflating. The first stage of recovery offers relief in this regard. We aren't going to try to unpack all of those feelings while we're just getting our feet moving on the mountain path. Once we're up out of the woods and into the scenic view, we'll have the strength, grace, self-care, and capacity to feel what we're feeling.

What Is Self-Study?

For the purposes of our recovery process, self-study is best accompanied by self-empathy. In the teachings of yoga, any practice that we choose to adopt gives us the opportunity to study ourselves. This is so because as soon as we make a commitment or adopt a new practice (drinking enough water to hydrate, going to bed on time, doing yoga breathing exercises), we get to see things about ourselves — how we respond, how we think about our new endeavor, when we feel like giving up — and experience an array of thoughts, reactions, and strategies that won't likely be unique to our newly adopted commitment. Likely these reactions reflect who we have been with ourselves, how we have talked to ourselves, and how we have given up on ourselves in the past. Because these glimpses of how we have been with ourselves can generate feelings of despair, disillusionment, or doubt, self-empathy brings kindness to self-study. Self-empathy reminds us we are experiencing the tribulations of the human condition. We are not alone.

With self-empathy, we approach self-study with openness, kindness, an eye for understanding, and an ear for tenderness toward all that we discover. Without self-empathy, we would primarily be studying the effects of the inner critic rather than learning who we are underneath our inner critic. Most of us have "examined" ourselves — we've thought and thought about why we do this or that; we've drawn up elaborate schemes to change our behavior, body size, or shape; and we've developed numerous ways to criticize ourselves under the guise of motivation, behavior correction, or discipline. But this is another reason why discipline precedes self-study: we need enough mental discipline to resist the inner critic and the inner "plan maker" long enough to genuinely learn about ourselves.

What Is Surrender?

Before we can talk about surrender in the yogic sense, we need to understand what surrender is *not*. Surrender is not resignation, nor is it apathy, though in our Western world it is associated with both. Rather, surrender, in the tripod of yoga, is the leg of the stool that reminds us not to become too rigid with our discipline nor lessen our accountability to our recovery with self-empathy's disguise: being "gentle" as an excuse to give up on pieces of our recovery in exchange for indulgence in old behaviors. Surrender is not used as a "reward" for maintaining the discipline and self-study required of recovery.

With yogic surrender, we surrender all distractions or interruptions that would prevent us from achieving our goals. We surrender harping on ourselves about our progress, punishing ourselves for setbacks, and indulging in self-recrimination under the banner of motivation. Surrendering self-hatred helps us stop our self-harming behaviors. Surrender becomes the doorway to self-forgiveness and freedom. Surrender releases old ways of behaving and thinking in exchange for new, fresh, and wiser ways of living.

 YOGA MINDFULNESS MOMENT

Discipline, Self-Study, and Surrender: "Going to the Bones"

Although it can seem paradoxical that yoga suggests both discipline and surrender at once, it is actually an incredibly elegant way to understand how we develop a healthy mind. We're going to explore this through a practice that I recommend you come back to again and again. It is extremely portable, always discreet, always available, very accessible, and it works!

- Bring your attention to the places where you now make contact, through the bones of your body, with your environment. Notice the specific sensations there, however subtle they may be. (At any one moment, the bones of your body are making contact with something in the environment. Heels on the floor, elbows on arm rests, shoulder blades on the bed or back of the sofa, hands on the steering wheel, or hips on a chair.)

- As you focus your attention there, you are practicing what we will label "going to the bones." You must use mental focus to do this. Stop reading and try this for one minute. In that minute, observe the effort required to consistently bring your attention back to the bones.

- As you practice this over time, through the doorway of focused attention (discipline), you will be more and more able to quiet your thinking mind. You will also become more aware of today's mental habits (self-study), and the need to resist (surrender) distractions in order to prioritize the mental focus of going to the bones.

I have instructed this practice thousands of times. It is always successful in that it brings us into relationship with the present moment. We will either experience the relief of the mindfulness intervention or become aware of how distractible our mind is. I personally use this technique frequently throughout my days and, at times, in the night. When I am awakened by a too-busy mind, I bring myself back to the quiet, tangible contact my bones have with the mattress or pillow, and I rest my mind there, ushering it away from anxious thinking.

Yoga: A New Lens through Which to Look

To really move into the possibility of yoga meeting the needs we've been substituting with food, we do have to shift the lens through which we have been looking for solutions. The teachings of yoga are a very different lens in two important specific areas: our cultural obsessions with gain-loss, pass-fail, win-lose, and deprivation-reward; and our cultural concepts of how change occurs (wherein failure is perceived as a lack of willpower and success is perceived as having been really disciplined and having made the "right" efforts).

The Deprivation-Reward Mentality

In the deprivation-reward mentality, we talk ourselves into deprivation techniques with the lure of a future reward; we overindulge with promises of future deprivation to make up for it. In the same moment that we decide to toss in the towel on a new behavior change, we've already committed to a deprivation strategy to make up for it. We toss our discipline to the wind because "we deserve [this indulgence]," yet, while we're tossing it to the wind, we're also planning our future reconciliation, also known as the "making up for it" activity. These internal agreements are the nature of disordered eating negotiations. And they reveal our confused relationships to discipline and reward.

In spite of its recommendations for discipline, yoga is not founded on a deprivation-reward mentality. The discipline of yoga, rather than setting us up for earned but not-so-healthy indulgences, directs us toward greater experiences of integrity, compassion, and steadiness. The discipline inherent in yoga has nothing to do with counting calories eaten and calories burned. It is not an evaluation of your body size, shape, or flexibility. Yoga is more concerned with how you live in relationship to your body, your vitality, your mind, and your community.

Let's consider some of the components of the deprivation-reward mentality: it is emotionally driven, occupies mental space, is disconnected from your body's natural appetites and your body's changing needs, is shame-based, is a reflection of fear, is time-consuming and steeped in black-and-white thinking, is intellectual rather than intuitive, and is unrealistic.

Looking through the lens of yoga will provide a very different but more sustainable and kind perspective. Yoga will teach you:

- how to live with self-respect
- how to become more intimate with your body's changing needs
- how to use discipline to lessen your unhelpful mental chatter (your inner critic)
- how to nourish yourself emotionally, spiritually, and physically
- how to develop greater intimacy with your appetites, needs, and desires
- how to cultivate discipline as an act of self-nurturance
- how to live in relationship to emptiness and fullness, physical hunger and satiation, and your emotional and spiritual appetites

Through the practice of yoga, you will have to steer your awareness away from the deprivation-reward mentality. Probably, you'll have to do this repeatedly. Consistently. Courageously. Because it's likely you've known this mentality for a long time, and it is so culturally driven that it shows up in myriad ways, not just with food. For example, notice how you relate to your "to-do list." Do you have to "get it all done" before you can relax? Notice how you fill your gas tank in your car. Do you wait until it's on empty, or beyond, before you feel willing to pull in to the gas station? Do you postpone doing things for yourself until other things, including other people, are taken care of? Does your self-care routine fall off your radar screen when life gets busy or stressful or when there are demands from other people? Do you consistently feel that you are "last on the list" of things you tend to?

If any of these is familiar to you, please know that you are not alone. And also know that steering away from this thinking will require courage and concentration. However, the rewards (pun intended) are worth it. To shift lenses to a yogic perspective on living brings freedom, aliveness, and integrity. In this environment, shame cannot sustain itself.

Creating a Skill Panel: The Sound Panel Metaphor for Recovery

Another important shift in lens that occurs via yoga is the shift to understanding how change occurs through a process that builds up specific skills while reducing our reliance on other strategies. We won't "win" by sheer force of more effort in an unskillful direction; and we don't fail because we "lack" willpower for change. We must engage in building new skills toward recovery while shifting away from shame-based, deprivation-reward, and all-or-nothing thinking. We must also simultaneously reduce self-harming behaviors to promote the healthy brain function that learns and integrates new things. This process can be called the "sound panel."

This metaphor has provided relief to many women trying to understand their painful food and body behaviors. In the midst of the pain, we have not known how to successfully turn toward recovery. More often than not, when we attempt to recover from self-harming behaviors, we approach the behavior, or set of behaviors, as the problem that needs to be controlled or eliminated. Thus, we end up struggling, with some futility, to try to change our painful behaviors. The sound panel as a recovery model suggests a remarkable shift in this thinking.

While making my yoga CDs, I spent countless hours at a recording studio east of Portland, Oregon. This studio had a very large sound panel with more than five dozen volume sliders, for adjusting and mixing a wide range of voices, musical instruments, and sounds. For the project I was doing, we used only two of these sliders. That was adequate for the specific task of recording the sound of my voice to talk the listener through a yoga practice. However, two sliders would have been entirely inadequate for recording a symphony.

Life is more of a symphony, both deserving of and demanding access to dozens of those volume sliders. We deserve a full range of emotional expression. We deserve access to our intuition, strength, playfulness, discernment, creativity, and passion (see fig. a.1 in the appendix). And life demands a wide range of social, intellectual, and physical capacities. Life demands intrinsic skills such as self-awareness and impulse control, self-attunement and discernment. Recovery is the process of adjusting our personal volume sliders to create a better panel of existing life skills, more harmonious interplay among our life skills, and enough volume that we gain traction in our recovery and harmony in our life. We can't get there just by trying to reduce our problematic behaviors or increase our healthy behaviors. It requires a balanced approach.

When we simultaneously reduce the volume of our self-harming behaviors and increase the volume of our new life skills, recovery becomes possible. Freedom becomes possible. Balance, joy, contentment, and ease all become possible.

If you've been using food and other behaviors associated with food, compulsive eating, body image issues, or yo-yo dieting cycles, you've created a distorted sound panel. Let's think of your main volume knob, your currently overused "survival skills" knob, as the one representing your disordered eating patterns, whatever those are, as a compilation of coping behaviors. The other volume sliders on a distorted sound panel can include things like overscheduling, rushing, or constant busyness; overachieving or underachieving; poor boundaries with self-care, with other people, or with work; self-perpetuating vacillations between pessimistic and optimistic thinking; self-defeating thinking; self-sabotage; and self-abandonment (see fig. a.2 in the appendix).

These are all generated as responses to, as symptoms of, disordered eating behaviors. Each one of these represents a strategy you've been using to try to manage your life, to fix your life within the bandwidth of what is familiar to you. That which is familiar has become your comfort zone, even if it includes painful aspects. When we try to journey toward recovery from within the vantage point of our comfort zones, we will not find success. But why?

- Because we'll be using the same mind that created the problems.
- Because we'll be limited to the sound panel knobs that we already know.
- Because it's still a search for control.
- Because we're doing problem management rather than new life skill development.
- Because some of our life skills to date are for control and others are for rebellion.
- Because our skills originally started as strategies to survive, to create a comfort zone in our early years, and we've outgrown that biological and social stage of our life.
- Because recovery is about creating your 360-degree life. Some part of you has a deeper urge for this than for a too-small (remember the 40 degrees?) comfort zone. And that part is very powerful! A lot of the friction we experience in our inner life derives from this more powerful urge for a 360-degree life.

With disordered eating patterns, the volume knob on the sound panel that relates to food and body strategies became the default setting. As we played this volume knob again and again, it became so overused, and overly relied upon, that all other possible skills (volume knobs) became unnecessary

᪐ Food has usurped our sound panel (see fig. a.3 in the appendix). Binge-ing and purging have overridden our volume sliders. Self-deflating inner talk has pushed our volume knobs out of balance in ways that we can't see, or hear, right now. And every time we turn to food, emotional eating, bingeing and purging, compulsive thinking, planning, eating, not eating, exercising, numbing, or coping, we push this one mighty volume knob way up. The other knobs become drowned out. Useless. Forgotten about. Weakened. Ineffective.

We've learned to use that one mighty knob over and over again. When we get sick of it, tired of it, despairing of it, angry at it, we think, "If I could just get rid of this . . . if I could just stop doing this . . . if I could just not hate myself so much for this . . . then my life would be better." While it's true that life will be better, more vibrant, more manageable, less painful, and less over-whelming when we are sober, this thinking won't get us there. Just getting rid of all of that with an attitude of hatred toward it won't work. Hating it is part of what keeps it in play. Hating it, we reach over and, with all our might, we pull that volume knob down. We push on it and push on it until down it goes and we wipe our hands saying, "There! Take that!" And when we turn our back, become less vigilant, become exhausted by the internal pressure, or get stressed by a feeling or an experience, the knob bounces right back up. Sometimes with more spring and power than it had before — a paradox-ical reaction to us having tried to hate it, condemn it, compress it down to a manageable volume.

(because we didn't need to develop them) and inaccessible (because addic-tion crowded out the ability to consider other skills).

In order to recover, we must simultaneously pull down the volume on dis-ordered eating behavior and increase the volume on the other knobs, the es-sential life skills knobs, which we will delve into in the next chapter.

To start on a recovery that will be truly different, a recovery based in yoga and all its wisdom, let's now acknowledge that our disordered eating behavior (1) started as a survival strategy; (2) developed into a coping mechanism; (3) provided relief, soothing, and direction; (4) became something we learned to rely on again and again; (5) grew to be our main life skill; (6) turned out to be so powerful that it crowded out our capacity for developing other life skills; and (7) led to the natural friction that happens when our old life skills no longer work.

When you take up the practice of yoga, you become your own sound master, as it were. And therein lies the hope that yoga will help you finally break free of your addiction.

3

CAPACITY
Four Essential Life Skills

FOR RECOVERY, YOU'LL NEED THE INFORMA-
tion that empowers you to hope, but you'll also need re-
newed and increased *capacity*. You're going to develop this capacity through
the building of four new life skills. These skills are presented throughout the
book intermingled with yoga exercises, breath work, and mindfulness tools. If
you've been battling with your body, you haven't likely turned to it as a tool for
learning. In the process of recovery, discovering how to learn *from* your body
will give you an entirely new relationship to your body and will teach you how
to develop self-care in the process.

Some of the tools of yoga that teach us to embody these life skills, or literally feel them and know them through our bodies, are *asana* (yoga postures),
pranayama (breathing exercises), and sensory-based mindfulness practices.
As a teacher, I prefer students learn life skills in a body-centered way so as to
have the life skill become embedded in the tissues, muscle memory, neurological response system, respiratory and circulatory systems, and mind. Integrating these systems makes it much more likely that when a situation requires
a response with a newly learned life skill, we'll be able to call on the corresponding synapses, muscle fibers, nerve endings, and cognitive patterns.

Fortunately, we don't need to learn a lot of yoga exercises in order for this
to be effective. That's because each asana, or physical pose, includes sensation,
body temperature, balance, strength, breath, mental concentration, and so on.
Any yoga exercise becomes an opportunity to learn from these components.

Let's explore how sensation, for example, helps us develop the new life skills we will be exploring in this book.

In your yoga practice, you'll learn to explore sensation as a body signal. Many people have learned to override or ignore some body sensations, such as thirst, fatigue, and even the urge to empty their bladder. Through yoga, we can open our relationship to sensation as a signal from our body asking for our attention. Then we might learn to identify a body signal, respond to it respectfully, experience the resolution of that body signal (such as quenching thirst), and learn how to tolerate body signals when we can't resolve them promptly (such as physical pain).

Similarly, another helpful life skill learned through body sensation is the ability to maintain openness toward our experience. Essentially, we're learning to stick with sensation in an open, mindful, and curious way. If you're like many people with disordered eating or body-centered self-hatred issues, you've already practiced reactivity, annoyance, fear, anger, frustration, or confusion in relationship to your body. Just think of the last time you got on the scale and were disappointed. Did you stay with the tender feelings of disappointment and grief, or bounce off to frustration, deflation, outrage, disgust, or despair? The ability to maintain open, curious attention toward a body experience — to anchor ourselves in the present moment and separate the experience of sensation from the story our mind tells us about the sensation — is a tremendous and courageous life skill.

Likewise, through yoga, you become more intimately aware of the nature of your thinking habits. Our brains can make developmental leaps when we train ourselves to transition from habitual, conditioned thinking to a fresh, open, and innocent way of thinking. Consider this simple life occurrence: driving to a familiar destination, like your grocery store. You probably have a specific way of doing this and some expected rhythm about it. If you change this up, even for one trip, you will experience freshness in your mind, your eyes, your driving patterns, what you see, and what turns you make. If you bring attention to this, you can see it all in a fresh and open innocence. You've just created a wider repertoire in your mind. And you have more knowledge about both yourself and the world. If you repeat this experiment, your mind will become more capable of opening its bandwidth in other areas of life as well. As you apply this to recovery, you will incrementally be developing a wider repertoire of life skills.

The four life skills we will explore in this book are (1) practicing grounding, attention, and presence, or what I will call "getting in the GAP" (this phrase may sound familiar to those who know Wayne Dyer's *Getting in the Gap*, but our work is unrelated); (2) getting comfortable feeling uncomfortable (GCFU); (3) moving from love, not shame (MLNS); and (4) increasing our personal buoyancy (PB). Let's look at each in turn.

Getting in the GAP: Grounding, Attention, and Presence

When it comes to food and body image, countless people are lost in a trance. The way any of us thinks about food, dieting, exercising, and our body shape is culturally ubiquitous, media-driven, and insidiously embedded in our culture's consumer mentality. Whether it's dieting or money, notions of gain, loss, reward, deprivation, accumulation, and fear are constantly reinforced. We don't need to have a clinically diagnosable issue with food or body image to suffer from the kind of thinking this milieu creates. Many of us are profoundly preoccupied with food, body image, weight, calorie counting, exercise, food as reward, exercise as redemption, restriction of food as progress or as "good" behavior, and overindulgence in food as "bad" behavior. Whether we experience this in mild or severe ways, the thoughts themselves serve a purpose. Understanding this purpose is key to helping us shift from this fixated thinking to the fresh thinking of recovery and to the journey of a 360-degree life.

What purpose could our culturally conditioned thinking milieu serve? It keeps us in a trance of mind that offers us (1) a *distraction* from other thoughts or life issues; (2) a sense of *belonging* to a cultural conversation (or compulsion); (3) an opportunity to get *control* over something in this otherwise uncontrollable, tender human life; (4) the illusion of keeping ourselves under control; and (5) a sense of *familiarity* wherein, like the veritable mouse in a maze, even though we are often confounded, the walls of the maze are familiar. Some of us are hopeful for a way out of the maze even while we hit our noses up against the walls of the maze's making. Repeated often enough, we fall into robotic, trancelike movements through our familiar maze.

Living an awakened and vital life, a 360-degree life, requires the precious and challenging process of extricating ourselves from this trance, from the maze itself, to lift ourselves into the wider horizons of well-being, freedom, clear thinking, and greater connection to our intuition and deep knowing. To lift ourselves out of this trance requires us to acknowledge the "benefits" that trancelike thinking has offered us. Part of our human nature longs for distraction, belonging, control, and familiarity — the rewards of the cultural trance. That there is genuine need being met by the trance is fundamental to how we address these needs. The tools within the practice of getting in the GAP offer relief.

Getting in the GAP is based on the yoga tools of focusing the senses (*pratya-hara*), mental concentration (*dharana*), and meditative awareness (*dhyana*), which are the precursors to freedom (*samadhi*).

Grounding: using our senses to get grounded in the present moment
Attention: wielding attention to cultivate concentration
Presence: becoming present through mindful awareness

Getting in the GAP lifts us out of the maze of ruminative or compulsive thinking, distraction, daydreaming, and dullness. Grounding, attention, and presence lift us into the space that exists between and beyond thoughts. In the GAP is the present moment, where we can experience relief from our brain trance, as we redirect our mind from its usual compulsive habits. In the GAP, we come to belong to our deepest presence, where we experience a felt sense of belonging. In the GAP, we experience refuge from cyclical, disordered thinking and a greater sense of control over where we put our attention. In the GAP, we cultivate a sense of familiarity with our native openness, where we experience clarity, freshness, love, and freedom.

At first, the practice of getting in the GAP will not feel as powerful as the cultural trance is in terms of fulfilling your needs for distraction, belonging, control, and familiarity. In part this is because the GAP experience will feel less familiar, making it automatically feel less accessible and reliable. Yet, truly, the process will ultimately be much more powerful for meeting your needs for distraction, which is really a desire to be free of our mental Ferris wheel of constant thinking. It will also more powerfully meet your needs for belonging and familiarity as you come to reconnect with your own center and discover the constancy of your own deep presence. With practice, the GAP process will become more powerful than the cultural trance that lures us with the illusory reward of control, as we learn to master where we put our attention and how we stay present.

The Trance of the Mind

When we live with addiction, compulsive thinking, anxiety, self-hatred, depression, lethargy, or persistent feelings of "not being good enough," we turn the trance of our mind into a painful biochemical and mental storm. We become both more anxious and more exhausted. Fresh thinking or new horizons are out of reach. We get trapped by the power of thoughts that pull us in familiar though unhelpful and often painful directions. These thoughts primarily center around attempts to gain some control and help us escape or manage our discomfort; they take the form of justifications, feelings of doom, castigations to work harder, or daydreaming, to name a few. Among these voluminous thoughts we may also hear competing thoughts. A thought of self-contempt might surface, triggering another thought of justification or a strategy to battle the self-contempt thought.

In this state, our mind is caught up in the trance of its own thinking. Most of the thoughts we have in this trance are repetitions of old thoughts, even though they have new names, dates, or events. These old thought patterns became the platform for thinking when we were very young, when our brains were developing, impressionable, and sponge-like. Even though we've grown and matured in many ways, some of our thinking is still tied to the past. Without our conscious knowing, the trance, while profoundly familiar, makes us tremendously vulnerable. We'll feel this vulnerability as the addictive strategies no longer work as well, or as they spiral out of control "for no reason." Yet the most important vulnerability is our fear of change. The trance of the mind is resistant to change and can perceive it as a fundamental threat. It's one reason that recovery can be so challenging. We want change; we even hunger for it. But when we make a bold new effort, after a certain threshold, something in our wiring keeps sending us back to our trance.

There is a second important consideration about this trance and our relationship to vulnerability: because these thinking habits and strategies were created to survive vulnerability, they're also programmed to avoid it. We learn to push aside vulnerable thoughts and become stronger than them. To avoid being vulnerable requires us to harden, to narrow down the realm of permission for what we think, experience, or feel. We become limited to the 40 degrees we've already known. Trying to push aside thoughts of vulnerability runs the risk of self-bullying. And it suppresses the opportunity to learn from our vulnerability.

Vulnerability:

Unskillful: causes helplessness, deflation, hardening against life or one-self; drains your capacity; causes isolation

Skillful: invites softness; allows us to feel the pain we've been in; creates a porous membrane through which new information and ideas can flow; and diminishes isolation

Yoga teaches us how to do this!

Yet, what about the idea that "avoid being vulnerable" or "push that aside and be stronger" might connote wise action? On the one hand, if we are continually made vulnerable by our own thinking habits, we want to reduce this painful process long enough to gain some buoyancy or resilience, long enough to remember that we're capable, valuable, and worthy of our own respect. Finding that "long enough" GAP is critical for recovery. Yoga creates these GAPs. The chronic thinking habits aren't capable of wisely directing us. They consistently send us back through the maze of long-held thinking patterns. We may try to overwhelm our destructive thinking habits with affirmations, positive thinking, or visualizations. Although these can be helpful, they'll be more powerful when paired with a deliberate effort to bring down the volume of destructive thinking. We bring down this volume when we learn to step into the GAP that exists between ruminative, compulsive, and habitual thinking, and our deepest knowing. That GAP is the silence between thoughts, even if it's only a split second. It is the moment of presence in which our mind glimpses a fresh possibility, a possibility other than the maze of painful, cyclical thinking.

This GAP essentially redirects our thoughts from the maze and gives us the opportunity to fill ourselves with fresh possibility and to reduce the vulnerability we are flooded with by our own thinking.

Key Elements

The GAP is the moment when we choose to step out of the trance of our thinking. The GAP lets us momentarily come into contact with reality, with our undistorted, actual self, with our capacity and potential.

GROUNDING
- Ground your mental focus to the physical, tangible present moment experienced in your sensory body.

- Use the more neutral (less internal, less prone to arousing thoughts of good-and-bad self-evaluation) sensory experience of where you make contact with the environment around you, such as being aware of where you touch the ground or the feeling of the air against your skin.

ATTENTION
- Repeatedly refocus your attention on the sensory experience; repetition will keep you tethered to the present moment and develops concentration.
- Practice this sensory attention moment to moment consistently. Even when your mind wanders, bring it back to the touchstone of grounding and pay deliberate attention to sensation.
- Practice this throughout the day to strengthen your ability to leverage this skill when needed.

PRESENCE
- Mindful attention toward sensory experiences deepens your sense of presence and refreshes your mind. As you practice, imagine your mind becoming refreshed through this process. This will increase the effectiveness of being able to return to presence more readily at other times.
- Presence through mindfulness is nonjudgmental; if judgment arises, drop back to the neutral sensory experience, such as the feeling of your hands holding the book.

When Thought Overwhelms Your GAP

We're tempted to feel obligated to our thoughts, as if they've been generated to help or guide or teach us in some way. Yet the maze of the mind produces thoughts from an older paradigm, the earlier life-survival paradigm. These thought patterns are taking up the space and brain energy that you could be directing toward your recovery. Some of them include black-and-white thinking, chronic self-evaluation, all-or-nothing thinking, self-criticism, self-abandonment, and the widely popular planning and reviewing. These thought patterns can become as tempting as certain foods. Getting in the GAP supports us in stepping out of these unhelpful conversations with ourselves. Here are some tools you can use to get yourself out of ruminative thinking and into the GAP:

- Become curious and affectionate toward your mental patterns. Rather than feeling obligated, annoyed, frustrated, or imprisoned by your thoughts, imagine the thoughts as being like old familiar visitors, impishly coming to torture you again. Pat them on the head and send them along on their way.
- Resist problem-solving the mental patterns. Stop trying to negotiate with your mind to think differently (it actually adds energy to the thought patterns).
- Learn to deliberately, repeatedly focus your attention on the tangible evidence of the present moment that exists beyond and in spite of thoughts. Consciously remind yourself that you belong to a larger life than any currently painful thoughts.

Getting in the GAP is a whole-person practice. It is mental, yet it also relies on the physical. It is neither suppression nor repression, though if you're strongly conditioned to believe that every thought you have is worth believing, examining, or negotiating, then this process may feel a bit odd because I am encouraging you *not* to follow your thoughts. This is not a passive practice. It is an active engagement with the fresh experiences of your sensory body. You are actively wielding your attention for the purpose of recovery.

✑ Feeling My Hands and Feet

As I put my attention more and more in my sensory body, as I am noticing my hands and feet, I am experiencing an amazing opening, softening, and surrendering. I realize that I have spent a majority of my life either running away from being in the present moment or trying too hard to force the present moment, thus staying in my monkey mind, restless, anxious, and distractable mind, never understanding what it was actually like to bring myself back to the present moment by noticing where my feet and hands are, throughout my day. In doing this practice, what is coming up for me is the awareness that I am not alone. My critical self is quieting. My thoughts are cleaner, softer toward myself and others, and I am paying attention and not going through life on autopilot.

—Kristen, age 48

YOGA MINDFULNESS MOMENT

Sensory Contact with the Environment (GAP)

Notice the way your hands are holding the book.

Feel your fingers on the pages or spine of the book, or the texture of your e-reading device.

Notice if some fingers are touching each other. Notice what your thumbs are doing and how they work differently but in tandem with your fingers.

Mentally make contact with where your feet are in your physical environment.

If you're wearing shoes, observe the feeling of your toes inside your shoes.

If your feet are on the ground, notice how they touch. Is one different from the other?

If your feet are up on the sofa, notice how they rest there.

If you are lying in bed, observe the weight of your heels against the mattress.

Notice the places where your skin makes contact with the air around you and the places where it doesn't.

Continue to notice as you read these words.

Now focus your attention on the sensation of your fingers.

What is happening with your fingers just now?

If your mind starts to get restless with this task, consider it an excellent time to practice staying with the sensory body as a place to get grounded. A restless mind is not uncommon in response to this exercise. It may even be a sign of how much resistance you have to getting present to the simple here and now, how little time you've spent doing it, or how unaccustomed your mind is to it.

Come back again to the felt sense of the pages or texture of the e-reader between your hands.

Notice the weight, the texture, or the feeling of this book or device intimately.

Let restless mind do its own thing and focus again on how your fingers are experiencing this present moment. Notice how they continue to experience a fresh relationship to the felt experience of the book.

As you keep pressing your thinking mind into the sensory experience of just your fingers, feel your mental state slowing down, your awareness opening up to a larger window of presence.

Notice that when your thinking mind is anchored to the sensation of your fingers, you are, for these moments, freer from ruminative thinking. Your mind becomes bathed in the simplicity of fingers holding the book.

Now, before transitioning back to reading, acknowledge any slowing down you've experienced through this short mental immersion into the sensation of your fingers. As you start reading again, if you find your mind gets busy and you lose track of any information or have trouble focusing, come back to the sensation of your fingers holding the book and refresh your mind again.

The Sensory Body

Our sensory body can only experience actual sensation in the here and now. Although we can remember sensation and even enjoy a memory, we can only experience the aliveness of sensation in the present moment. In this way, our sensory body can be used as a grounding tool.

Most of us have become accustomed to not fully engaging with our sensory experience. Although we may favor sensory experiences that are pleasant, the practice of getting grounded is not dependent on pleasure. The practice of getting grounded in sensory aliveness acknowledges that all sensory events are temporary, ever changing, and fresh.

Most of us were not taught to engage with our senses to understand life. We weren't shown how to awaken our awe to the coolness of a dip in the lake on a hot day, or the feeling of the grass, or the way the temperature of the bathwater continues changing as we sit in it. We may have been taught to notice how pleasurable these experiences are. But usually we weren't taught to immerse ourselves in the sensory experience for awakening our relationship to our body. We may not have been made aware of how ever-changing the sensations of the body can be, or how normal this is in certain situations. We didn't develop our sense of nuance for sensation, but rather we developed a more superficial relationship to sensation, one that set out to determine whether the sensation was good or bad.

The human organism longs for a felt sense of life through our senses. It connects us to nature and to life beyond our own thoughts. Not having sensory training can mean we'll struggle with managing sensations that are uncomfortable. Learning to be in relationship to neutral sensation is how we will start to develop the skills we need to move toward the uncomfortable sensations and the uncomfortable experiences of life. The next essential life skill for recovery, getting comfortable feeling uncomfortable, focuses on just this task.

Getting Comfortable Feeling Uncomfortable (GFCU)

Whether or not you have an addiction, a compulsion, or a confused relationship to food, if you are like most people, you don't like feeling uncomfortable. We don't like feeling physically uncomfortable, mentally restless, or psychologically overwhelmed. We're disinclined to invite or enjoy a stubbed toe, a migraine, disappointment, panic, frustration, or helplessness. Rather, we're inclined to avoid, resent, or prevent these things.

Although human organisms are programmed for specific biological imperatives associated with survival, we're also designed for spiritual imperatives associated with evolving. One imperative wants to protect us, which it will do through adrenaline, defense mechanisms, and strategies to avoid pain. The other wants to encourage us, which it does as we live into the life skills of surfing discomfort long enough to learn that we won't die and that we can keep trying. For example, we don't remember teething or learning to walk, yet we know that both of these childhood experiences included plenty of pain on the way to capacity. Clearly, we didn't give up. We grew through those experiences.

Yet, as human beings, since we do have hardwired programming to avoid discomfort and seek comfort, we've learned to associate avoiding physical discomfort with our survival. For example, our biological system is programmed to avoid too-cold or too-hot temperatures for the safety of our vital organs. We have programming that regulates our body temperature by retaining body heat or by sweating. We don't have to think about this for it to happen. We're also programmed to produce biological responses to threat, such as a fever in response to an illness or a throbbing pain in response to stubbing your toe. These responses are the body's way of protecting itself from further harm and alerting us to danger.

We can also transfer physical discomfort to psychological discomfort. For example, let's say you have a response to caffeine like I do: you feel shaky and your heart races. You drink caffeine and then go to a social function. Your heart is racing from the caffeine, but this also mimics physical symptoms you have with anxiety. At the gathering, people make jovial conversation with each other and you perceive them as overlooking you. Your heart races a bit more and you start assessing yourself as uninteresting. Then you may actually feel physically anxious. How will you spend your time at this social gathering? Your breathing goes up into your chest and you start looking around for the best place to be a wallflower. You can't believe this is happening to you again. You knew you should not have come to this party. You are always a loser at parties. Now you're also experiencing the cascade of perceived-threat programming (fast heart rate, shallow breathing, thirst, heightened body temperature, and so on). As you find your place to isolate yourself and wait out the uncomfortable social gathering, you wish you had gotten some water. Now it feels too exposing to walk over to the beverages and get some water. What if someone wants to talk to you?

In this scenario, a physical sensation induced by caffeine prompted certain responses, which prompted thoughts, which prompted your survival mechanism (that is, to isolate yourself). If you can hold on to your sanity enough to realize that the caffeine induced the first sensation and your thoughts started going haywire, you might be able to rein in your anxiety.

Although the hardwired response to discomfort is embedded in the human organism, for the purposes of survival and of regulating the body, it is the competing urge to evolve that makes your quandary with food a cause of so much suffering. Addiction, compulsion, and related strategies start as attempts to protect ourselves, but ultimately they block our ability to evolve. That means that the pain you're feeling today is the necessary pain for your evolution. The pain you're feeling today is the pain of countless compressed previous pains you didn't have the chance to learn from. In this regard, today is a day to celebrate. Discomfort is your invitation to grow in ways you could not have previously considered, until now. Getting comfortable feeling uncomfortable is the first step toward pain as an opportunity to outgrow the pain you have been in.

This will require several paradigm shifts for you:

- Discomfort is an invitation to grow.
- Addiction was once a useful survival tool that now blocks your evolution and causes devolution.
- Avoiding distress is akin to avoiding your potential to grow.
- Short-term relief adds to long-term stagnation.
- Getting comfortable feeling uncomfortable lets you explore your growing pains with curiosity.

- Getting comfortable feeling uncomfortable opens you up to the possibility of a 360-degree life.

Even though disordered eating patterns ultimately became very painful and made you miserable, one of their greatest advantages has been giving you the ability to avoid distress and to override discomfort. Disordered eating gives us the illusion of having some control (albeit short-lived) over whether or not we feel comfortable at any given moment. This is also one of the greatest disadvantages of an addiction. Once we've programmed a behavior to bring on a degree of relief from our discomfort, it's very hard to give it up. At the point that you're at right now (you've picked up a book about the subject) the struggle to give up painful behavior can be very baffling, because you aren't getting deep relief anymore, what relief you do get is always temporary, and it's now also accompanied by a lot of pain and misery. Yet those few degrees of relief are painfully seductive.

In recovery, we'll have to get comfortable feeling uncomfortable, but not only in the sense of feeling things that are painful. We'll also need to learn to get comfortable feeling joyful, confident, radiant, and so on. Surprisingly, the unfamiliarity of these feelings is often among the more uncomfortable discomforts!

Getting comfortable feeling uncomfortable is the process of learning to tolerate small discomforts by mindful effort to feel your body, heart, mind, breath, and environment. It is the process of observing the distress as it arises, welcoming your physiological response to the distress, and then getting more comfortable with the sensations. It is also the discovery that all feelings and sensations pass; they are temporary messages to become present to yourself.

When you are uncomfortable or distressed, accompanying physiological sensations alert you to the discomfort. Even if your primary discomfort-avoidance programming is in thought, you will still have associated physiological sensations of discomfort *before* your discomfort-avoidance strategy comes on line. Once we've used a substance or an activity for a certain period of time, even the thought about the substance brings on feelings of relief. Therefore, in recovery, it becomes helpful to identify the discomfort-avoidance strategy as not just the physical act of reaching for food, weighing yourself, or going for a ten-mile run. The thought that precedes the behavior is a part of the cycle. For example, prior to a thought about chocolate cake, a new diet, or isolating yourself at home with ice cream and a movie, your mind-body is uncomfortable about something. Often this uncomfortableness is an accumulation of discomforts. Yet when our getting-comfortable-feeling-uncomfortable skill hasn't been developed, it won't take much accumulation for discomfort to trigger our compulsive programming. Some of the tools we gain through yoga include increasing our ability to feel our body's sensation signals sooner and lengthening our ability to withstand the discomfort long enough to open a window of possibility into new responses.

Therefore, relearning how to experience discomfort comfortably, without trying to manipulate, solve, control, or suppress it, is one of your essential skills for recovery. I'll also suggest that at some point you will be grateful for the symptoms of discomfort; they become your yellow flags of caution (by the time something is a red flag, it can be too late). You may even find you are able to respond curiously, lovingly, humbly for the opportunities discomfort presents. There is deep learning in recognizing that we experience a specific discomfort and, without us trying to push it away, manipulate it, or override or deny it, it passes and we survive it.

GETTING COMFORTABLE FEELING UNCOMFORTABLE

The Step-by-Step Process

1. Getting in the GAP provides the foundation for getting comfortable feeling uncomfortable. Using physical sensation, we tether ourselves to the present moment and observe the nuances of sensation.
2. To start with a nuance that is safer to feel, begin at the level of your skin and work inward toward your muscles. Observe sensations slowly; acclimate to each layer as you go. Imagine yourself as if you are in a glass submarine moving slowly down through the ocean; there is much to see and take in.
3. When you land on a place of particular discomfort, such as a tight muscle, pause. Ground yourself (still the submarine) at the area of the sensation. Bring your attention to the sensations.
4. With respect and curiosity, explore the sensation. Become present to what your body offers you in the inquiry.

5. Then move the submarine a bit more deeply into your discomfort and observe how your breath moves in relationship to the discomfort.
   - Is it shallow? Tight? Choppy? Smooth?
   - Is your breath located more in your chest or in your abdomen?
   - Does your diaphragm feel pliable or stuck?
6. As you stay with your experience, become aware of any urge to analyze, manipulate, suppress, deny, amplify, discharge, or medicate your sensations. Get very still and watch what your mind is doing in relationship to your discomfort.
   - Does it jump, dart, hide, attack, act suspicious, become hyperalert, or dash away?
   - Does it move in close, hoping to conquer the discomfort?
7. While kindly but actively resisting your mind's urges, calmly note to yourself that you are surviving the physical and mental uneasiness in a tangible moment-to-moment way. Your discomfort may not be greatly changed, but you are coming into relationship with yourself and with your discomfort.
8. In this relationship, you will begin to feel more comfortable around your own discomfort. You will be opening your window of tolerance for discomfort.
9. If necessary, repeat to yourself: "I am learning to get comfortable feeling uncomfortable. I am, moment to moment, surviving this terrible discomfort. I am expanding my capacity in life and growing an essential new skill."

YOGA INQUIRY

Getting Comfortable Feeling Uncomfortable (GFCU)

Here is a chance to practice.

Lie on your back with your knees bent. Using a yoga strap, keep your left foot on the floor and bring your right foot into the strap and stretch your leg up into a hamstring stretch.

Relax your breathing softly into your abdomen and before you let your mind become distracted by your hamstrings, bring your awareness to the more neutral sensations of this experience:

Notice the way your left foot is making contact with the ground.

Notice also how your hip bones, shoulder blades, and head make contact with the ground.

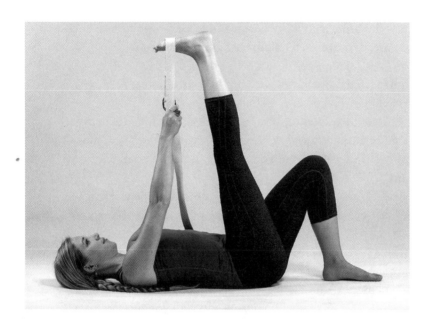

Identify these as the foundational elements of your pose and also as places where your mind can become connected to neutral sensation.

Then observe how your hands are holding the strap. As needed, loosen your grip so there is no unnecessary tension in your hands.

Allow your breathing to soften again and prepare to bring your attention to the next layer of sensation: your hamstrings. As you notice your hamstring stretch, I invite you to slowly move your leg a bit left to right and to research a place where you feel your leg can be still for a couple of minutes. Then ask these questions:

- Do the sensations have a particular shape?
- Is there an associated temperature?
- Is there any texture to the sensations?
- Do they have a color? Is it dense, cloudy, or transparent?
- Are the sensations smooth or bumpy or changeable?

Notice these intricate sensations.

You may also observe a mental response: reluctance? curiosity? something else?

Keep noticing the experience of sensation. Maintain the intention to withstand your mental chatter about sensations and get to know the direct physical experience.

Are the sensations fluctuating? Is there nuance to how your muscles or bones are responding?

Notice any response you have in your abdomen. Does your breathing shift? Do the muscles of your belly have a response?

Notice any arising sense of impatience, confusion, or resistance.

Equally notice any arising sense of curiosity, intrigue, or acceptance.

Open to the possible array of feelings that may arise.

Stay with this for three more breaths.

With mindful attention, release your right leg and repeat this exploration with your left leg up in the strap.

This same concept could be practiced with mindfully exploring a cool wind against your skin or standing in the rain just past your threshold for enjoying these experiences. Notice that these activities are centered on body sensation. And, in all of them, you have some control.

Physical sensation can become discomfort that takes you by surprise mentally. Likewise, psychological and mental discomfort will always be accompanied by physical sensation. Addressing tangible sensation is an act of courageous intervention. We're willing to feel what we feel. And, in feeling it, we're also slowing down our psychological, perceived-threat programming.

Making Ourselves Uncomfortable

With food addiction or food disorder, there are countless ways to produce our own discomfort. Below is a list of some of the more familiar ones. As you read the list, read slowly and attempt to *feel* your body-mind response. Some of these will be more familiar to you than others, but try to feel each one and the capacity it has to bring on discomfort.

1. Getting on the scale; even though it could produce a happy outcome, it is chronically linked to an unhappy relationship with your body and most often it produces disappointment; even if the number is one that relieves you temporarily, it is always short-term relief
2. Eating past the point of fullness or until you feel bloated
3. Restricting your caloric intake until your head spins, your stomach aches, and your body and mind are exhausted

4. Compulsively exercising to the point of physical pain
5. Believing you are supposed to be a certain size and shape and weight, and feeling profoundly disappointed for every perceived small and large flaw
6. Pulling the covers over your head and remaining depressed and lethargic in bed
7. Having unscheduled free time that turns into bingeing on food, TV, Internet, and the like
8. Overusing laxatives
9. Determining good foods and bad foods, and then setting yourself up with far too few food choices to feel safe in the grocery store, at a restaurant, at a family meal
10. Eating in secret, from the garbage, or in hiding and feeling ashamed of it
11. Being too near to foods that are triggers for you, such as meeting friends at the bakery instead of the park
12. Repeatedly upsetting your blood sugar levels

Someone who does not have a food- or body-loathing-related compulsion might just tell us to *stop* doing these things. Yet we've tried that! It wasn't so easy. Somehow, as baffling as this can be, we're compelled to do things that actually cause not just discomfort but also harm, self-deflation, and misery. This is primarily because the "other discomfort" we're in is too hard to manage, and these ways of being uncomfortable offer not just a bit of the familiar discomfort but also enough momentary relief to keep being compelling.

Building Resilience

During the process of recovery, we'll have to work with discomfort that is arising in the here and now, such as a headache, a physical craving, sleepiness, or the discomforts of hunger, a properly full stomach (if you've been a restrictor), or a just-full-enough stomach (if you've been a binger). At other times, we will experience discomfort that has been suppressed by the years of our behavior. These could be both wonderful and disquieting experiences, such as feeling expansive, open, and alive and not knowing how to be with that, or feeling the underlying anxiety that food has been pushing down for you. We won't be able to avoid this en route to recovery, but applying getting-comfortable-feeling-uncomfortable tools will certainly help.

Additionally, it can help to understand a few things about our discomfort tolerance and our resilience (the section on personal buoyancy, on p. 66, will discuss resilience in more detail):

1. Some of this programming is genetic. People are born with greater or lesser capacities for resilience.
2. Resilience, at the level of the brain, is moldable; it can be reduced, but it can also be increased.
3. Every time you run the same course, the programming gets stronger and more ingrained.
4. Every time discomfort is something to be avoided with food or other behaviors, it is more likely to demand that from you next time.
5. Every time you don't run the same course, the programming is weakened, and you start to have options where you didn't previously.
6. Every time you get comfortable feeling uncomfortable you strengthen your ability to do it again and again. This is the essence of resilience.

Moving from Love, not Shame (MLNS)

One of the ways we've unknowingly learned to make ourselves the *most* uncomfortable is through the voice of our inner critic. I can tell you with great conviction: your inner critic has nothing new or intelligent to offer you, does not have your best interests at heart (and never will), and cannot be trusted to help you with the spiritual imperatives of your recovery. Your inner critic is designed to keep you safe, but miserable. It is designed to make sure you don't take risks, and therefore stay captive to old ways of doing things. And it is fundamentally interested in being right about you, from a terribly narrow perspective: the perspective that you are flawed, that you need constant monitoring, and that you need to improve yourself in order to gain acceptance and love. These are the ground rules for shame. To free ourselves from shame, we must cultivate new ground rules, ones based on love. Love, in this regard, is how we express self-kindness, tenderness, and accountability. Moving from love means orienting from self-kindness and respect for your human journey. Making this switch will require you to look at your life through a new lens.

Many years ago when I was in art school, we were given specific assignments to open our creativity. In photography, we experimented with different speeds of film, with shooting from the hip, and with developing processes in the darkroom. Most exciting, we experimented with making our own cameras and lenses. We were being encouraged toward discovery, toward widening our options, toward breaking out of our box. The process that we will call "moving from love, not shame" is like shifting the camera lens. It is a deliberate act of rebellion against the voices of shame and an intentional shift to love, self-respect, empathy, forgiveness, tenderness, and faith in yourself.

One of yoga's fundamental teachings is that our basic nature is love. Love is experienced as a felt sense of belonging, deep contentment, abiding ease, and joy. It is an overarching feeling of acceptance, inclusion, warm welcome, and understanding. In love, we experience profound tenderness and affection toward all that is and has been. Love is expressed as innate respect and care for our body, mind, and heart, and for our thoughts, actions, and relationships. Love allows us to feel what is precious and fleeting, without fear of the ephemeral nature of all things. It allows us to move fiercely toward truth, and it requires us to uphold integrity, passion, and fervency in the face of harm, or threat of shame. Love is the force through which any sense of inadequacy is burned away, allowing the blazing clarity of our deepest worth to shine forth.

One of addiction's fundamental misunderstandings and messages is that we are deeply and innately flawed, that we are shame itself. Shame is the profoundly painful feeling of believing that we are essentially inadequate, broken, or not worthy of belonging. It is a sense of never being good enough, no matter what. Shame is the feeling of being beyond inclusion, beyond repair, beyond ever proving ourselves otherwise. It is an insidious and invasive force that feeds our critical inner voice, our constantly condemning inner judge, or our anxious and fearful mental radar screen. It keeps us scanning the environment for threats, walking on eggshells, or striving ruthlessly for perfection. Shame is also our apathy, our waterlogged sense of futility toward life's possibilities. It is in the muscles of our giving up, and in the subconscious grip of our resistances to change.

Addiction manifests through the lens of shame, and, through the processes of addiction, we continue to mistake our basic nature to be shame. Through this lens, we live with the impossible task of trying to overcome what we deem to be flawed, unacceptable, or broken. This impossible task requires so many resources from us, and is so powerfully seductive that we've unknowingly reduced our options down to managing shame, which keeps us in constant negotiations with shame. Exhausted by this constant negotiation, we give more power to shame and forget that we can shift the lens ourselves.

The Development of Internalized Shame

How did shame become so deeply embedded and overwhelmingly capable of overshadowing our innocence, joy, or beauty?

In the earliest years of life, our mind-body is extremely porous. At sea in a kind of osmotic membrane through which we expressed our physiological needs (for food, warmth, contact, and so on) to the world around us, we were also constantly taking in that which surrounded us. We soak up the environment we're exposed to, including the facial expressions, gestures, and feelings of our parents, caregivers, siblings, or community, and the ambiance of safety, chaos, nurturance, tension, depression, optimism, and so on. Because we're born with the right hemisphere of our brain being dominant (the left hemisphere does not come on board promptly), we swim in this sea of osmotic experiences in which we feel everything as us. If we cry and a human shows up, we experience contact. When we giggle and the other humans giggle, we've made an impact on the world. Equally, when someone in our environment is angry, despondent, overwhelmed, or anxious, we experience that as an extension of us. If our giggle can cause others to giggle, perhaps we also caused the rage, despair, anxiety, or sense of being overwhelmed.

As we go on soaking in this sea of experience, if we are swimming in a primarily invalidating or misattuned environment, we're being slowly deprived of our capacity to retain our innocence, native joy, and unbounded expression as love itself. What makes an environment invalidating may be as "subtle" as an unstated but felt sense that a parent or caregiver is chronically disappointed in us. It may be as overt as physical, emotional, or sexual abuse, all of which infiltrate to the most vulnerable core of who we are. Abuse from persons who have more power than we do, particularly when they have responsibility for or control over our survival, causes profound confusion, powerlessness, and pain that can become debilitating later in life. Another way invalidation occurs is through being consistently blamed for other people's feelings, frustrations, or circumstances.

Because we're programmed with a deep longing to be seen and mirrored, which is critically essential to our sense of security in the world, being in an environment in which who we are in our uniqueness is a disappointment, is invalidated, is regarded as not good enough, or is impossible to celebrate for parents who may be distracted by their own life events makes us profoundly vulnerable to internalizing this invalidation. We experience "There must be something wrong with me; and despite my efforts, I am helpless to change it." If this overwhelms our system enough, the shame we internalize obscures our innate radiance and sense of belonging. Ultimately, we learn to operate from a base stance that we are, essentially, shame. We learn to regard ourselves in some of the same painful ways that others regarded us. We invalidate our own needs and feelings. We criticize or condemn ourselves.

While we've been trying to manage shame, we've unknowingly been strengthening its hold on us. It is absolutely essential and tremendously powerful that we shift from managing shame, where the primary orientation is that *it* is more powerful than *us*, to living in relationship to it, where *we* are more powerful than *it*. Because shame has been so insidiously internalized, even a shift to living in relationship *to* it, rather than *from* it, represents a shift in the power balance between us and shame. Our first step in this process is acknowledging that shame exists. We acknowledge that shame has invaded the place in us in which our basic worth would normally reside and that it has infiltrated our mind and body. Our vigilant reorienting to love must be practiced through radical acceptance, empathy, and a willingness to experience our vulnerability and our strength, with faith and constancy, especially when shame arises.

The practice of yoga gives us the tools for reversing the internalization of shame. Through the practices of asana, pranayama, and meditation, we directly and intimately experience the truth of our being as worthy of love and belonging. When shame has repeatedly overwhelmed love, we'll need a tool more powerful than shame to recalibrate our physiology. Because yoga has the ability to affect us at very deep levels, it is our more-powerful-than-shame tool.

At the root of all addictions lies a deep well of shame. At the heart of all recovery is the healing power of love.

Moving from Love, not Shame: Key Elements

RECOGNIZING THAT SHAME EXISTS
Shame is more of a force field than an emotion. It is insidious, palpable, and sticky. It is the ruthless force of the inner critic. Once you begin to see how it has been infiltrating your own psyche, you will also see it in others, in family systems and cultures, and in media and advertising.

Shame can disguise itself as a helpful, motivating voice; yet no one has ever learned brave new skills from shame. We can feel shame in ourselves, and we can feel it for another being if we witness them being humiliated, painfully rejected, abandoned, or banished. When we live with inner shame, these are our own chronic fears, too.

Shame tells us not to take risks, not to let ourselves off the hook, not to let go of control, not to forgive ourselves for our imperfections, and not to see our bravery, beauty, and tenderness. Shame is our internal bully, the kind of person we would not enjoy being near if he or she existed on the outside of us as a breathing human being who spoke to us the way we speak to ourselves through shame.

FEELING THE PHYSIOLOGY OF SHAME IN YOUR BODY

The feelings of shame can include a hot fire in the body, thirst, heart palpitations, cold sweat, dizziness, sudden onset of a foggy mind, hypervigilance, racing mind, sudden fatigue, feelings of powerlessness and isolation, and so much more. We'll know when we've entered the shame field because our physiological system will tell us. Sadly, most of us haven't learned to respond to this system with real first-aid skills. It's as if the fire alarm is going off and rather than looking for the escape route, we're running toward the fire while tossing fuel on it with our thoughts. Or, by contrast, we might seem to be frozen in place by the power of the belief that we deserve to feel as terrible as shame makes us feel.

Your body will register these physiological sensations in your specific patterns of response to threat. Learning to feel this as a physiological alarm is an important step in learning how to move from love, not shame. Mercifully, yoga also teaches us the tools to forcibly shift ourselves out of shame and back to love.

FOCUSING YOUR MIND AWAY FROM THE MENTAL
BROADCAST OF SHAME

When shame is present, it threatens to take up the entire viewing screen. It wants to prevent us from seeing anything other than shame. When this is occurring, if we give in to the broadcast, it will get louder. In our early stages of recovery, we can use the tools of getting in the GAP or getting comfortable feeling uncomfortable. This might include the feeling of your feet on the ground or the pages of a book in your hands. It can include the sound of morning birdsong or traffic outside your window. If we turn our attention to only the tangible, neutral, sensory experiences of the present moment — by getting in the GAP — shame cannot be as much of a bully.

USING THE GAP TO GLIMPSE *LOVE*, NOT SHAME

This GAP lets love and belonging reenter your body, your heart, and your experience of life. Grounding, attention, and presence afford us a mental, physiological, and visceral opportunity to shift from shame to love as we get a glimpse of stability, connection to life, and the felt sense of belonging.

OPENING TO THE POSSIBILITY OF
NOT COLLAPSING INTO SHAME

When we practice getting comfortable feeling uncomfortable, one of the greatest advantages we'll have in life is more power over shame itself. With this skill set, we won't have to collapse into shame's spell. When we use our skills to feel the physiological rush of a shame storm, a rush of windy thoughts, torrential emotions, and physical sensations, we dissipate shame's power. When we're willing to turn toward ourselves rather than shame, shun, or condemn ourselves, we gain power over shame. Not collapsing into shame supports our journey to our 360-degree life. Not collapsing also means we're not left out of the circle of our own belonging, and we can let love in. Love, in this case, is the simple, moment-to-moment willingness and attention we're giving to ourselves through mindful awareness.

REMEMBERING THE COUNTLESS OTHERS
WHO ARE AFFECTED BY SHAME

Actively remembering the countless others who have been impacted by shame ends our isolation and generates empathy and compassion. Even if in the beginning we aren't readily able to offer ourselves empathy and compassion, most of us would offer it to another person suffering under a shame storm. Offering this either to ourselves or others will also expand our capacity to move toward our 360-degree life. Empathy and compassion for others can act as life vests in a shame storm. Eventually, we'll be able to bring ourselves into the heart of empathy and compassion.

TETHERING YOURSELF TO LOVE

As you practice these steps, you will find a kind of automatic programming start to take over where your previous auto-programming to shame was taking up mental space. It won't feel mechanical or contrived, and it won't take the same amount of mental effort to move through these steps. Rather, you'll find that as a shame storm sets in, your auto-programming will shift to moving from love. The good news is that you will feel this shift washing through your mental, physiological, emotional, and physical pathways. Where shame used to run these currents, you'll be opening up to love to fill these riverbeds. This is the process of learning self-care, self-respect, self-attunement, and self-love, all of which are available to us through the practice of yoga.

YOGA INQUIRY

Shifting Posture, Shifting from Shame (MLNS)

Body posture can invoke certain feeling states. When we slump on the couch there is a particular mind-body-emotion field that we slump into. Before you think it is the couch that causes that, consider that curling up on the couch with a book is a very different mood. Likewise with standing tall in arrogance, or standing upright in your integrity or openheartedness. Think about how your body responds when you experience shame. For me there is always a component of contraction. In contrast to that, think about how your body responds when you feel generous, compassionate, or loving. For me there is always a component of expansion.

Taking on the physical characteristics of a particular mood or emotion is one of the ways that we learn what something feels like. In fact, we learned most of our facial expressions from watching those around us in our very early years. Actors and actresses take classes on movement and facial expression to learn to feel what they need to exude in playing their characters.

This yoga practice is not meant to be a resource for you only when you are in a shame storm. Body posture and expression has been embedded over many years. To shift it requires us to practice in both times of threat and "non-threat." This is a simple, very portable practice. And a very powerful one!

You can practice this while you're reading, but I also want you to practice it when you're standing in the kitchen, walking through the grocery store, or in your seated meditation. Bring your attention to your body and your breath. Inhale deeply and exhale with a little sigh to clear your heart. Then let your attention come to your heart or the region in the center of your chest. Very slightly lift your sternum (the bone in the center of your chest) and your collarbones. Imagine this like taking the lid off the top of your heart. With this lift, welcome the inner experience of expansiveness and allow it to flow from your chest outward, in a quiet gesture of inner confidence, generosity, and tender care for life, including yourself. Also, with this lift, allow the kindness of life to flow back into you. If you haven't experienced much kindness in life, imagine it like the rays of the sun or the feeling of a warm breeze. Neither the sun nor the breeze chooses to shine on or touch only specific people and things. They're both unconditional. The shade of a tree is like this, too. Its comfort is offered to all.

Take five or six conscious breaths with this intentional inner expansiveness. Let the experience soak into you, the way a sponge soaks in the ocean.

Before returning to reading, or any other activity, acknowledge that posture has power, breath has power, and mental attitude has power. Shame has had a lot of power over you. It's time for you to have some power over it.

INCREASING PERSONAL BUOYANCY (PB)

In the processes of recovery, we will need enough buoyancy to tolerate the discomfort and challenges associated with change, to prevent ourselves from backsliding, to give ourselves the courage and stamina to keep going when life is overwhelming or when we feel vulnerable and unsteady in our recovery, and to steer clear from shaming ourselves in the process of the very normal ups and downs of recovery and life. Personal buoyancy is your float-ability, your bounce-back-ability, your resilience, and your ability to maintain or regain your sense of hope, faith, and courage when your recovery feels vulnerable. It is supported by a healthy enough physiological state, clear thinking, foresight, self-care planning, and the other life skills we've been discussing.

As with the large exercise balls we use at my yoga studio, which require us to reinflate them from time to time, your personal buoyancy needs you to take care of it because it is affected by all aspects of your life, including the stages of your recovery (it becomes easier to maintain the longer you are in recovery). It is impacted by how much and what kind of use you require of your brain, body, heart, and vitality in the course of a day, a week, or an hour. And your base genetic makeup also contributes to your innate level of resiliency.

Your "personal buoyancy factor" (PBF) — a term I use to help us talk about the measurability of our personal buoyancy — is tangible. You have already felt this. Some days your PBF is really low, while other days it's higher. You

~✒ Shame Monster and Bingeing

Last week I watched myself get seduced into a binge. It was very strange because I really didn't even want to do it. I was aware of my robotic movements but couldn't seem to connect to them. Even during the binge it felt like "work." Then I did something new. I stopped midway and threw away the food. I didn't want it. It was making me feel sick without any of the payoff. Later I reflected on how or why this happened. What did I not pay attention to? Then I remembered honestly revealing (briefly) to a new friend on Wednesday that I had a history of an eating disorder. I didn't elaborate or even over-reveal. But still it was a risk, and I remembered the fear I felt afterward about many things. What would they think of me? Now they would know deep down how crazy I am. I had had an encounter with the shame monster. Instead of directly acknowledging her shame monster presence, I think I tried to deny her existence. I think this really had a lot to do with my binge.

—*Allison, age 42*

have had experiences on one day that cause you to binge miserably; on other days, the same experience doesn't fluster you into a binge. You've seen friends have an experience in which they became agitated, yet you know you would have responded very differently. And you've had ups and downs that would not have flummoxed someone else. When we start to think about the variables in our fluctuations as influenced by the measure of our PBF, we can become less vulnerable to blaming or shaming ourselves for our ups and downs. We also become able to work with our PBF to help prevent the unnecessary down spells.

Recovery will require you to make changes in your life. Specific changes will raise your PBF greatly, including targeted changes related to body image, food, compulsive eating, and yo-yo dieting. If we attempt to put new concepts into our life without changing the parts of our life that contribute to our addiction, we'll be swimming upstream with new swimming strokes, but against the same currents that exhaust and threaten to drown us. Recovery will be much more powerful, more sustainable, and a lot more fun if you learn to protect and promote your PBF with the new skills you are learning.

Understanding Your Personal Buoyancy Factor

There are two physical activities that I have done that required supplemental oxygen: scuba diving and hiking at high altitudes. With scuba diving, we wore air tanks to deliver oxygen to our scuba masks and to our lungs. With high-altitude hiking, we trained at lower elevations first and acclimated ourselves to the gains in elevation we anticipated for our journeys in Peru and parts of Utah. How much oxygen a person used in her scuba tank was a matter of how conditioned her lungs were, her breathing rate, and the duration of the dive. How much training a person needs for high-altitude hiking is a matter of what elevation he lives at, the condition of his lungs, the amount of cardiovascular exercise he already engages in, and his prior experience at high altitudes.

Much like both of these examples, your PBF is the result of your innate (genetic) resilience; your early life experiences in calm and nurturing, chaotic and invalidating, or unpredictable and painful environments; the amount of time you've spent "in training" with the other tools we've explored; and the wear and tear imposed on you by your daily life. Although we can effect change at the level of our genetic resilience, we can't change it like flipping a light switch. We also can't change the early life environment we lived through. An area we do have capacity to add to our personal buoyancy includes enhancing our life skills tool kit and addressing the wear and tear of daily life. The reciprocity of this system makes it personally rewarding and increases the likelihood of us wanting to nurture and reinforce our PBF.

If you've had to pump up a bicycle tire, you know that there is an optimal amount of air pressure to put into the tire. In this same regard, there is an optimal personal buoyancy factor for you, and an optimal way to think about how you maintain your PBF. To many of us with addictions or disordered eating strategies, we've grown accustomed to thinking in black-and-white, good-and-bad terms. We might be extra disciplined, careful, stern, and holding steady, albeit to a fairly thin line. Or we might be all-out bingeing and chaotically pushing out against our rigid deprivation mode. While these are understandable urges for (and struggles about) control, this mind-set will not produce personal buoyancy, nor will it actually produce the desired outcome of control.

Tending to your personal buoyancy will require a sensitivity that isn't possible with black-and-white thinking. Black-and-white thinking promotes reacting rather than anticipating, observing, tuning in, and responding. When we're stuck in black-and-white thinking, we miss critical opportunities to do things differently, to learn a new way. The practice of personal buoyancy invites us to anticipate, to practice foresight, to tune in to our buoyancy factor, and, based on self-awareness and respect, to respond in favor of recovery. Throughout this book you will be introduced to concrete ways that you can specifically nurture your personal buoyancy. You will see this in chapter 4 ("Fervency") as "Reasonable Guidelines for Respecting Your Body Intelligence and Nourishing Your Life Vitality," in chapter 5 ("Finding Faith, Reviving Courage") as "Unearthing Faith: Creating Personal Buoyancy through Self-Accountability," and in chapter 6 ("Resilience and Self-Empathy") as "Getting in the GAP: Your Body Dashboard." At this juncture, we're going to focus on the deep mental rest your mind needs to help you with your recovery.

Deep Rest for Your Mind

One of the biggest causes of diminished personal buoyancy is exhaustion. Arranging your schedule to support you in getting deep rest, real rest, is a critical component of your PBF. This deep rest is critical to your recovery because recovery itself will require clear brainpower. When brains are developing, as in the stages of human development from infancy through adolescence, the human organism needs a lot more sleep. (Just look at how much babies and teenagers sleep!) The same is true of a medical crisis where the patient is put into a medical coma, or when a person has undergone a surgery of some kind and sleeps more during the rehabilitation process. It's not just the hip that needs to heal from a hip surgery. The entire body is recovering, and resources have to be allocated properly for recovery. You also know from personal experience that it is harder to enjoy activities, learn new skills, and maintain clear thinking when you are mentally exhausted. Therefore, arranging your life to support your deep rest and rejuvenation is critical to your PBF, and thus, your recovery.

Below are some suggestions for supporting your mind to get deep rest.

- Schedule your life to allow you to get a proper night's sleep.
- Reduce rushing, urgency, and haste.
- Reduce how much unnecessary stimulation you expose yourself to in the course of a day (e.g., Internet, media, advertising, social time with overstimulating conversation, and so on).

- Balance your schedule to allow for downtime. Create white space on your calendar.
- Set boundaries around what kind of social events you go to, how long you stay, and what you'll eat. Decide this and commit to your boundaries before you arrive.
- Toss out your scale.
- Cancel your subscription to fashion or beauty magazines.
- Reduce how many hours of TV you expose yourself to on a daily and weekly basis.
- Turn off or walk away from your cell phone for a period of time every day.

◆ YOGA INQUIRY

Creating White Space (PB)

Culturally conditioned thought patterns, deprivation-reward strategies, and old thinking styles crowd out your mental "white space" and cannot help you recover. Yet these mental patterns will all arise, as they've been doing for some time, and they will be more tempting when your mind is exhausted. Accumulating periods of white space promotes your brain's ability to reset itself to crave this reprieve, and to be renewed more promptly, too.

In a sea of doing rather than being, thinking rather than feeling, and reacting rather than responding, most people's schedules, lives, and brains are too crowded. White space is the unplanned space on the schedule, the open space in the rhythm of your life, and the unengaged space in your mind through which grace can enter.

To create white space in your day requires you to plan ahead and hold fast to your boundaries. To create white space in your life requires you to tend carefully to the rhythms of your week, your month, your season, as well as your personal needs for renewal, your family's needs for structured and unstructured time, and the unexpected detours of illness, stress, or life events. In the beginning of recovery, white space can be terrifying. Therefore, we practice it in increments. Here's how:

Set a timer for specific increments throughout the day. This could be once an hour, or at particular intervals that represent transition (waking up, leaving the house, arriving at an appointment).

Set a minimum of five opportunities for this.

When the timer chimes, create a deliberate pause of one minute.

Take a few deep breaths to release what you were doing.

Then do nothing. Sit still. Observe. Witness. Feel.

On day two, repeat this but increase it to two minutes.

On day three, increase it to three minutes.

Make this your practice for one week. That will add up quickly to more than an hour a week!

You may experience a variety of things during these mini-meditations. You may need the skills you have developed for getting in the GAP, getting comfortable feeling uncomfortable, or moving from love, not shame. The accumulation of this habit will reteach your brain how to rest and will reawaken your mind and body's craving for rest as a tool for your health and wellness. Without white space in your brain, your day, and your schedule, you will be perpetually engaged with mental strategies, planning the future, reviewing the past, and stirring old thought habits.

In time, I would like you to build your comfort with white space to create thirty minutes a day, several hours a week, and eventually whole weekends of white space. We can't discover new strengths in ourselves if we don't have the white space in which those strengths can surface. In this white space, it isn't that nothing is allowed to happen. Rather, it is a strategy to structure your day for a time-out that lets you choose renewal, check in with yourself,

❧ Mini-Meditations

Today has been a good day for me — so far. I started the day listening to the guided meditation with legs up the wall. During the day I'm honoring my intention to complete my mini-meditations every hour or so. And this has really helped my ability to, while in a toxic work environment, return to center and remain nonreactive to the swirl of emotions that have become a norm.

— *Theresa, age 44*

and be available to something spontaneous that can nurture your recovery. Many people have forgotten how to allow for wise spontaneity. Recovery requires a kind of thoughtful spontaneity in which your refreshed brain can evaluate its personal buoyancy to determine how much it can "spend" and what it needs to "preserve."

 YOGA MOMENT

Savasana (PB)

During recovery, you'll need a proper amount of rest for your body to recover from the onslaught of metabolic and digestive issues related to eating poorly, overeating, and overdieting. Add to that enough rest for your brain to metabolize the changes you're going through and the developmental leaps you'll make as you follow the practices in this book, and deep rest becomes a time for profound recalibration. An important aid to deep rest is the yoga pose called *savasana*.

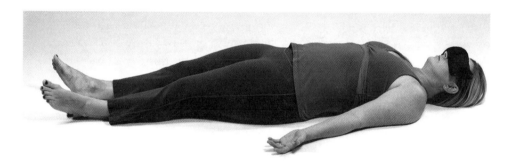

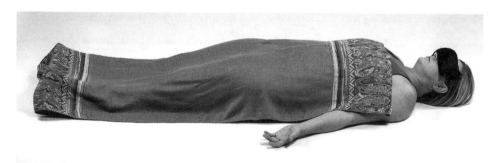

Savasana is commonly the last pose in a physical yoga routine. It is a pose of rest and integration. Savasana is done by lying on your yoga mat and simply resting. You can tailor it to be more personal and nurturing.

1. Set a timer for twenty minutes. Make sure the timer sound is not startling.
2. Use an eye pillow to quiet your eye movement, which also quiets your mind.
3. Cover yourself with a favorite blanket, shawl, or scarf. I use my favorite sarong for this because it's not too heavy for the summer and travels well.
4. Although silence is preferred for this ritual (and easier to travel with), you may play soothing music.
5. Lie down and allow yourself to become very still.
6. If your mind is busy, use this mantra: Just Rest. Just Rest. Just This, Deep Rest.

Part Two

SELF-NURTURING
DISCIPLINE
(STAGE ONE)

4

FERVENCY
Desire and Discipline

Tapas, the first stage of recovery, is based in discipline. "Oh, great! I could really use more of that!" you might say to yourself. Or, "Now, we're getting down to business here. Enough about mindfulness and rest. What I need is discipline!" In anticipation, you may want to hurriedly read forward through these next few pages looking for a new strategy for getting control over your "lack" of discipline. Although you will find solutions here, I caution you not to search these pages for that one new trick. That thought process itself keeps us looped into the cycle of disordered eating. What you'll read here offers you the chance to open up new relationships to discipline and desire. This chapter outlines processes for finding healthy ways to experience both. It takes discipline to embark on this journey—a fiery discipline that actually transforms, not a discipline that sets us up to fail or reinforces hopelessness.

Tapas, or fervency, is defined as: (1) the fiery transformation that arises from the friction of discipline, (2) a fiercely loving, intense commitment to self-awakening, (3) constancy in effort toward the goal, and (4) the foundation of your 360-degree recovery.

You'll find that in Sanskrit one word can have several related translations. The word *tapas* translates not only as "discipline" or "austerity" but also as "heat," "purification," and "transformation." I like to translate it as "the fiery transformation that arises from the friction of discipline," or "fervency." This friction is the friction between what we know we most long for—freedom—and our overused coping mechanisms, which block us from our freedom. It is the friction between our desire to be healthy and our rebellious self. It is the friction between our deep knowing that each episode that occurs within the cycle of addiction only perpetuates our pain and the predictable, instant relief (albeit short-term) of indulging in our behaviors. It is the friction between self-nurturing discipline and self-hating discipline. It is the friction between that to which we say *yes*, and that to which we must say *no* in order to live into the *yes*.

From a yoga perspective, the fervency of these frictions leads to transformation. We can't transform one substance into another without rubbing the two sticks together to generate the fire for transformation. When we aren't able to use our will — our ability to leverage direction and fortitude from ourselves — to generate the commitment for the effort, we'll either remain stuck in our cycle of personal despair or we'll go numb. It's very hard to start a fire with waterlogged wood. We can't transform our overused coping mechanisms into self-loving discernment without the fire of effort and discipline. As painful as our inner frictions may be, through yoga's path to recovery, we will come to know them ultimately as the frictions that catalyze us to transform our lives. Someday, on the other side of the pain, we will know the meaning of grace. We will come to thank pain for requiring us to recover, to recover our whole self, as it were — to come back to life. But to navigate this recovery, we will need the fervency that this yoga path demands. The fervency of our longing for freedom and wholeness, to which we say *yes*, must overwhelm our fevered reliance on our self-harming coping mechanisms, that to which we must say *no*.

❧ YOGA MOMENT

Breathing Intervention — Saying No *to Say* Yes

1. Stand in horse stance. Step your feet two to three feet apart, with your toes turned out slightly and your knees bent.
2. Firmly plant your feet.
3. Stabilize your legs and pelvis.
4. Make your hands into fists.
5. Rotate your torso and let your arms swing, twisting left and right, while your fists strike the back of your waist and sides of your ribs. Let the weight of your arms support the pace of the twisting motion.

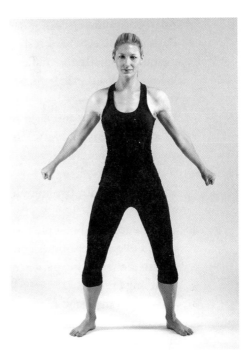

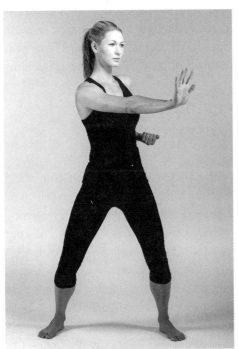 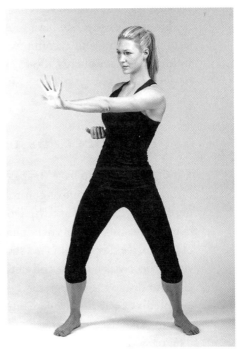

6. After one minute, twist more vigorously and shift to "pushing hands." Pushing hands is a hard gesture that emphasizes the heel of the hand pushing out, much like the traffic cop signaling STOP.

7. With a vigorous exhale through your mouth, push the heel of your hand out.

8. With each exhale and each push of your hands, mentally say *no* to that which threatens to overwhelm your recovery, such as a thought of your own, an internal storm, a criticism from another person, a brownie calling you from the kitchen.

9. Stick with this for two minutes, exhaling vigorously. Make the entire two minutes count.

10. At the end, stand completely still and feel the waves of aliveness in your body. Follow your body's craving for a deep inhalation. Deliberately connect to the sensory experience your body moves through in the echo of the breathing exercise.

11. As you feel that echo in your body, say *yes* to your aliveness — *yes* to your belonging — *yes* to your capacity — *yes* to valuing yourself enough to stay on course.

Note: Sometimes you'll have to "act as if" you feel strongly enough to say *no*. Sometimes you will have to exaggerate the vigor in your exhale to more strongly express your commitment to yourself. Amplify the intensity of your feelings to "move energy," de-fog your mind, or push away feelings of lethargy or doubt.

THE PENDULUM OF DESIRE AND DISCIPLINE

For those of us who have struggled with disordered eating, we've known the turbulent swings of out-of-control desire and discipline. We've been driven by desires, fought against and hated our desires, and punished ourselves for giving in to our desires. On this pendulum, when our food issues swing painfully out of control we desperately seek strategies to "get ourselves under control." Discipline becomes punitive and steeped in self-loathing. At times it seems that to give our discipline enough momentum, we rev up the insanity, so that we are essentially at our very worst, "hitting bottom" as it's sometimes called, before we can "take the swing" to the other side. Swinging back and forth between longing and coping, between unhealthy desire and unhealthy discipline, will not lead to recovery. It painfully entrenches us further and profoundly limits us from experiencing lasting freedom.

If you're reading this book, you've probably lived this pendulum. On one side, the pendulum swings toward compulsive, painful behaviors, robotically, even feverishly pulling us along a trajectory we've come to know all too well. On the other side, the pendulum swings toward our desperation for this to end. By increasing the punishing deprivation or atonement strategies, we hope for relief. When we're frenzied enough by this cycle, some part of us comes to deeply believe that it generates our conviction for recovery. We might even tell ourselves, "The more desperate I become, the greater my conviction will be." Tragically, this swinging pendulum only serves to perpetuate the cycle.

Yoga's path holds that recovery is possible when we loosen our grip on this pendulum. To do this, we must understand the underlying tensions of our relationship to both desire and discipline, and we must create new relationships to both.

Desire

Disordered eating causes us to struggle with confusing, painful, and conflicting desires. For example, we may desire nourishing companionship but turn to ice cream for solace instead. We may desire purposeful work, but turn to bingeing for self-soothing, even though it leaves us numb. We may desire radiant health and vitality but compulsively seek control through rigorous self-denying diet rituals. Our desires for nourishing companionship, purposeful work, and radiant health, to name a few, are not bad, nor are they problematic. Even more critical to know: these desires are not unrealistic. In fact, these are the intelligent desires of our life force. This life force is the vitality that wants you to thrive, to be vibrantly healthy, so that the life that is best meant to come through you can. Much like the force that enables birds to take flight and gladiolas to bloom, this life force has a unique expression through each of us. Underlying this life force are the intelligent desires that prompt you to come to life.

The predicament is that ice cream, bingeing, and rigid diet rituals, though painful, provide just enough relief, and quickly enough, that our deeper desires get supplanted. We divert ourselves, again and again, with things that have historically provided more immediate solace. Turning to food has made sense because it's readily available, it produces biochemical responses of satiation and reduction in anxiety, and we know how to do it. However, by repeating these behaviors, we have essentially programmed our minds and bodies to be able to robotically initiate and complete our food, diet, and exercise rituals. And when the behavior is practiced enough, even the thought of the ice cream solace that we will reward ourselves with at the end of a difficult day is enough to provide immediate relief to our brain and body. Similarly, the thought of tomorrow's workout to burn off the calories of a compulsive indulgence provides just enough permission and fleeting sense of control that we feel we've strategically, and safely, bargained for the binge (and arranged for it to have as little impact or lasting evidence as possible).

Our robotic, immediate-relief strategies, in action and in thought, soothe us in dangerous ways. In addition to greatly reducing our ability to tolerate discomfort, these strategies also flatten our desire "landscape." Our conflicting desires become merged with each other in our mind. How did this merging occur?

The Merging of Desires

Our brains take time to develop. In early life, we cry because we are hungry, cold, wet, tired, overwhelmed, or lonely. We aren't able to discern these experiences as the source of our impetus to cry. (Sometimes our crying baffles the adults around us, too, as they try food, diaper changes, naps, and playful attention to soothe us.) Similarly, when our brains are in early development, we may register a feeling of hunger, but underneath we're lonely and don't know how to identify it. Slowly, through experimenting and experiencing, we learn to identify needs and satisfy them naturally.

Those of us with disordered eating patterns had this natural process interrupted. We came to believe that our physical signals were bad or wrong, that our base desires were problematic or overwhelming (first to others, but then internalized as overwhelming to us, too), or that something about our desire was dangerous and could not be trusted (if our innocent expression of desire or need, for example, overwhelmed a parent's parenting ability, or became cause for them to feel frustration to the point of shaming or harming us). Quite likely, we were raised in an environment in which we didn't learn how to tend to our body's unique way of signaling these needs and desires, as well as our body's unique way of announcing its satiation of these needs and desires. We came to internalize messages from our environment, took cues from grown-ups, and experimented to find out what we could safely feel and what we ought not to feel.

Because this occurred at a time when our brains were tremendously malleable and subject to the kind of shaping that becomes reflexive, it's not surprising that we bring certain behaviors forward with us as we mature into adulthood. Although we're twenty or more years older, we still instinctively turn to certain foods for solace. We've grown up and become more capable of complex thinking, but our earliest self-soothing strategies, because they were successful in providing relief (albeit short-term) and went unchallenged, remained intact. This can be quite confounding to our now more grown-up intelligence! We see ourselves moving through the robotic pattern of our food, diet, or exercise rituals and know we should not be doing it or wonder why we are compulsively doing the very things that exhaust us or drive us to anxiety and depression.

Because we have come to label our compulsive behaviors as "bad," unearthing what our deeper desires might be gets lost in a sea of badness as we, without even identifying those underlying desires, lump them into badness itself. After all, it is those desires that produce this bad behavior, isn't it? To the part of our brain that has not advanced with our biology, this thinking makes sense. And so we merge the badness that we feel about these painful rituals with "by association" badness toward our deeper desires, the very ones that represent the intelligence of life trying to pull us forward from suffering to vibrancy.

Another painful and unforeseen outcome of our reliance on these self-soothing strategies is that we've greatly reduced our ability to tolerate discomfort. We've programmed ourselves to need immediate relief. We have not had to learn how to withstand the discomfort of our desire for nourishing companionship, for example, nor how to tolerate our loneliness. We have not learned how to tolerate the inner conflict between our deep desire for radiant health and the overwhelming messages of self-hatred and never-good-enough that keep us detached from the innate loveliness, and lovability, of our own bodies. Unknowingly, our robotic, immediate-relief techniques have prevented us from having the opportunity to grow in these ways. In our repetitive reliance on immediate relief, our ability to leverage our discomfort for learning and discovery has become profoundly atrophied. The good news is that, like the muscles of the physical body, the practices of yoga also develop and strengthen the suppleness of our life muscles for self-awareness and for tolerating discomfort.

᭤ Recovery will require us to practice getting comfortable feeling uncomfortable in all areas of life. Truly, life requires it. So you might remind yourself that every step you take in recovery is also a significant investment in your life as a whole. Your 360-degree life will require that you get comfortable feeling uncomfortable, in both unpleasant *and* pleasant experiences. It may surprise you to know that many people struggle with the discomfort of feeling extraordinarily good, radiant, or content. Simply said, they don't know what to do with themselves. At times, in recovery, it is feeling tremendous that may become the trigger for painful behaviors. Therefore, we use the skill of getting comfortable feeling uncomfortable (GCFU) in all stages of recovery and to prepare ourselves for what life feels like when we aren't in constant pain.

We do this using one of the essential life skills discussed in chapter 3, getting comfortable feeling uncomfortable (GCFU).

Getting Comfortable Feeling Uncomfortable: Just for This Moment

Giving yourself permission to truly feel what you feel, to experience what you experience, can cause you to feel uncomfortable. If having permission to feel what you feel wasn't offered to you in earlier life, giving yourself this permission now can feel unsettling, like you are breaking a rule or about to get into trouble. If you resist feeling what you are feeling because you are afraid it will last forever and be too painful, know that you are not alone, and that this is a sign that this fear has been trying to protect you from feeling for a long time. Discovering that feelings and experiences are occurring just for this moment helps make opening up to feelings safer and more manageable. Going to the thoughts of "forever" and "too much" are requests from your brain and body to move more incrementally when you're in the realm of bigger feelings.

"Just for this moment" is the process of seeing what is, feeling what is, noticing what is, and acknowledging it as our experience just for this moment. We're staying current rather than suppressing or denying, both of which result in stored or postponed experiences and feelings. When we bring our attention to and actually experience body sensations, acknowledging that this is indeed what's occurring, just for this moment, we begin to get comfortable feeling.

YOGA INQUIRY

Just for This Moment (GCFU)

Let yourself become still and quiet. Relax your face, your jaw, and your breathing. Become aware of the temperature in the room and any peripheral noises. Then bring your attention to a body signal, something tangible and evident in this moment. When you're ready, spend a minute on each of these:

- I'm feeling [this body signal (achy muscle, droopy eyes, thirst)]. I accept that this is a sensation, a signal, a symptom my body is producing—for this moment.
- Just for this moment, I do not need to override my body signal. What I am experiencing is legitimate, changeable, and temporary.
- Just for this moment, I do not need to alter my experience. This body signal is a valid expression of the human body, my body.
- Just for this moment, I do not need to dismiss my experience. All on its own, this body signal will continue to change.
- Just for this moment, I do not need to suppress what I feel. I can courageously admit, without any shame or guilt, that this is what I am experiencing right now.

All of our body signals—in fact, all of our mind-psyche-emotion signals—are expressions of the complexity of what it means to be human. We have experiences that impact us. We accumulate our experiences in our body, in our mind, in our emotions. An expression, at any one moment, is both a vital reflection of who we are, including the influences of the culture we live in and the experiences we've had, and an ever-changing, nuanced, fleeting expression. A muscle ache may be the result of mental tension, poor food choices, or a new or more strenuous activity (to name a few things). It is the vital expression of the whole. A muscle ache also has subtle fluctuations within it. Observing the fluctuating nature of sensation reminds us that this is what is happening just for this moment.

As we learn to observe how body signals and mental broadcasts influence each other, such as when a thought of anger toward the body for having a muscle ache increases tension in the body, we will gradually come into awareness of how we generate a mental train of reaction to get away from, resist, avoid, medicate, or manipulate our experience. This is where we'll greatly benefit from the skill of getting in the GAP to help us navigate a nonreactive relationship to what is occurring.

Getting in the GAP: Mindful Attention

Yoga tells us that one-pointed attention is one of the greatest tools to overcome suffering. How could that be if what we need to pay attention to is an area of pain or confusion? The act of paying attention is one slice of what our mind does. It is the slice of attention that happens before we're reactive, before we feel dread or elation, before we collapse into despair or get clouded in by disappointment. It is the moment that notices what simply *is*, before we add our likes and dislikes. Of course, over millions of brain interactions, we've taught ourselves to experience our mental "train" as a sequence of information that turns into reaction. The practices of yoga give us the chance to slow this down and take one small incremental slice at a time. In this first act, we're just learning to pay mindful attention. Mindful attention is open, nonjudgmental, nonreactive, and reflective, the way a mirror objectively reflects objects, and it offers us clear information to which we can respond, rather than react.

This process of getting connected to information is very similar to the way our cellular phones get connected to the signal that makes their reception clear and usable. The information we connect to through paying mindful attention is more usable than our reactions are. Reactions create the biochemical rush of anxiety, resistance, frustration, or deflation, and in those storms, it's very difficult to use the information clearly.

Paying attention to your body-mind-psyche is an empowering, connecting, and courageous opportunity. It grants you the opportunity to feel, discover, learn, and grow. Not paying mindful attention only offers us more of the same, more of what we already know, much of which is not working that well for us. Keep in mind that as you start to pay attention to the signals from your body-mind-psyche, you may initially feel frustrated if you don't know how to respond to those signals. Many people ignore, override, or dismiss their body's signals (desires). You are having an opportunity to re-learn this yourself now. Identifying what you feel is the first step toward learning how to wisely respond to what you feel. At this stage, I encourage you simply to try to pay attention, openly, nonjudgmentally. It is an act of valuing the thing to which you give your attention. Therefore, be aware of that to which you give your attention: Is your attention on real-time, body-centered sensations or on the mental broadcasts of fear or the sense of being overwhelmed? This is a foundational step along the journey of re-learning how to choose what we are valuing and how to wisely respond to our body, our feelings, and life at large.

YOGA MINDFULNESS MOMENT

Mindful Attention: Increasing Our Ability to Value (GAP)

Because I'll ask you to commit to staying hydrated as a demonstration of your commitment to yourself (in chapter 5), you will have several opportunities every day for this practice:

- Get yourself a glass of water or pick up your water bottle. Prepare to use water for mindful attention.
- When you pick up your water, notice the shape, texture, temperature, and weight of the container it is in. We rarely pause to notice these nuances, yet we constantly experience them and our brain constantly calculates appropriate responses. (That's why when you pick up a glass of water, you don't spontaneously splash yourself in the face with it.)
- When you sip your water, acknowledge its value to your body. We're made up of 57 to 60 percent water (on average).
- When you sip your water, pause to feel the experience of water in your mouth: notice its temperature, weight, and texture.
- When you sip your water, feel the act of swallowing the water and follow the sensations of the water going down to become absorbed into your body.
- When you sip your water, mentally reflect on this act of self-care as an expression of your personal value, to yourself. Feel the body sensations that arise with this reflection.
- When you sip your water, for every time you pay mindful attention, you are increasing your ability to value yourself.

Many of my students use the moments of sipping water throughout the day like a meditator might use a mindfulness bell. It is, quite literally, a moment of refuge, a moment of self-value, a moment in which they remember they're on a path committed to recovery. (Some will use water-sipping mindful attention during meetings, business responsibilities, social engagements, or homework marathons to remember to keep themselves and their body on their radar screen — in their attention span — for recovery.) As you become experienced with this one, you will be able to translate this mindful attention practice to other body signals: the urge for a few moments of rest, the experience you have in falling asleep at night, the feeling of your skin warming up in the shower and saying "yes."

A Balanced Relationship to Desire

When you apply the tools of yoga to your recovery, you will unearth an entirely fresh relationship to desire. Once you come to live in a balanced, non-harming relationship to desire, it becomes as natural, as non-self-denying, as turning on a light in response to dimness or closing your eyes to listen more exquisitely to birdsong. Through yoga, you learn to respond to desire with curiosity, patience, and permission. In the beginning, this may be a steep learning curve — at times joyous, at times frightening. Therefore, during early recovery, we are more methodical. As your recovery grows, you will come to innately respond to desire with celebration, and you'll recognize desire as one of the ways life's intelligence expresses itself through you.

BODY SIGNALS AS DESIRE

In Abraham Maslow's famous framework for understanding the hierarchy of our needs, physiological needs form the base. When healthfully tended to, our physiology provides a stable foundation from which we can attend to our other innate needs. Included in his model are safety, love and belonging, and esteem. With those levels of need stabilized, we are able to move toward the top of the needs hierarchy: self-actualization.

Establishing a healthy physiological base requires tending to our body's signals, satisfying the preprogrammed and biologically driven needs for breath, food, water, rest, and homeostasis that sustain us as an organism. Unfortunately, those of us who have dis-regulated our body's physiology will find that we don't know how to tend to those signals, or that our body is giving us confusing signals, such as mental fatigue and food cravings. Furthermore, compulsive behavior dulls our ability to inquire into our body's signals, and urgency to satisfy the compulsive drive overwhelms our capacity to stay engaged with more nuanced body signals. Immediate-relief behaviors prevent us from listening long enough to hear our body clearly and limit by many degrees our 360-degree life. Yoga provides a framework to live in an intelligent, responsive, and balanced relationship to desire, beginning with cultivating sensitivity toward the signals of our physical body. Yoga heightens our ability to listen to our body's signals and brings us into attunement with our body, where we have access to a concert of sensation through which to inquire about our body's messages.

Yoga also teaches us how to respond to our desires in a timely but nonurgent manner, much like acknowledging the fuel light on the dashboard of the car. When the fuel light comes on, we neither go swerving feverishly through traffic to screech up to the nearest gas pump nor do we drive on for miles until the tank is empty and we are stranded at the side of the road. Although we don't generally ignore the fuel light on the dashboard of our car, we have countless times ignored the warning lights on our physiological dashboard, dulling our ability to acknowledge and wisely respond to it.

When our relationship to desire has been infused with confusion, guilt, or shame, it is critical that we establish a fresh relationship to desire itself so that we can come into balance. To begin this conversation, I propose this as a working definition of *desire*: a sensation experienced in the physical body that alerts us to an underlying need. This underlying need may be rooted in the physical, emotional, or spiritual layer of our being, and is accompanied by sensations in the physical body. These sensations motivate us to explore the satiation of a desire. Much like water satiates thirst, empathic companionship satiates our need for belonging. We experience both of these satiations in the physical body. In moments of all-encompassing satiation, all layers of our being experience profound contentment. In this state, we are free from anxiety, shame, and fear.

Notice that the base definition of desire is neutral. When it is free from shame or suggestions of "badness," desire is a natural, healthy, biological drive. Even our drives for belonging, esteem, or integration are programmed into our being. Yet those of us with disordered eating patterns became profoundly disconnected from the innate intelligence of our body. Sadly, we live in a culture that perpetuates this as normal, even admirable. The fact that this arrangement has turned into painful disordered symptoms is, on the one hand, a gigantic pronouncement from your body that this *does not work for you* and, on the other hand, is a blessing in disguise. From a yoga perspective, your body is trying to get your attention on behalf of your mind and heart:

❦ Quick Reference on Body Signals as Desire

- Because our relationships to thirst, hunger, fullness, rest, and movement have been confused, using tangible body sensations — experiences that are touchable, feel-able, and knowable — to relearn how to identify desire, and the satiation of desire, is necessary and helpful. To experience this embodied knowing is invaluably empowering.
- Learning to attune to these sensations as signals of desire begins with learning to bring mindful attention to sensation in the body.
- Once we learn to feel body signals nonreactively, openheartedly, and mindfully, we can transfer that learning to our ability to identify our thirst, our hunger, or our need for rest, proper exercise, fresh air, and so on.
- To whatever we are giving our attention, we are also increasing its value. Valuing our body's sensations may be a new frontier, yet is much more life-giving than repeatedly valuing shame's messages.
- In the process of allowing for attention and attunement, we will observe that sensations come and go. We will learn that desires come and go. Discomfort comes and goes. We will learn to get comfortable feeling uncomfortable (GCFU), using our "just for this moment" tool, and learn to trust our body's signals.
- Sensation is a healthy process of our body's moment-to-moment experiences. Desire is a healthy response from any biological organism, arising in relationship to its inner and outer environment. Through acknowledging what is occurring, we acknowledge to ourselves that our body signals are valid, informative opportunities for discovery, growth, and evolution.
- The ever-changing, ever-arising nature of desire can feel overwhelming. In the beginning, you may think, "How will I ever keep up with all of this?!" With a tangible, body-centered approach, it quickly becomes easier to stay in the moment-to-moment experience, where life is more manageable and less overwhelming.

this agreement to disconnect from the innate intelligence of your body does not work for you. The friction you experience within this is the blessing of your fervency. Without the friction, you'd be unlikely to seek solutions, to seek transformation.

Later in this chapter you'll be offered a yoga exercise to help reawaken your ability to feel your body's unique way of expressing sensation, producing body signals for you to wisely, curiously, respond to, and to stretch your ability to explore openheartedly the acceptability of how your body expresses desire. You will be invited to know your body's signals as valid, intelligent representations of reasonable needs and desires. The process of inviting, feeling, and responding will stimulate a reawakening of your body's ability to produce honest signals for you. If you have been disconnected from yourself, to some extent, this reawakening may include feelings of tenderness, grief, or poignancy, the sorts of feelings people have on journeys of homecoming. You may also experience troubling feelings. As we reawaken an area of our body-mind-psyche that has been dulled, we occasionally bring to light old feelings that we were not able to safely experience as they were occurring.

Earlier in this chapter I suggested we initiate this process methodically. In this light, I suggest that if emotions arise during your yoga practice that you acknowledge them like you might a song on the radio in the next room, but keep your primary attention on sensation in the body with a focused, neutral, and open attitude. There is a time for you to work through more troubling feelings as your recovery progresses. At this juncture, it's important that you don't get derailed from the process of reconnecting to your body's signals. This discernment requires your deliberate practice, and it will empower you to identify your desires for thirst, hunger, rest, proper exercise, fresh air, and so on. You will observe that sensations come and go, that desires come and go, and that discomfort comes and goes. Experiencing the natural ebb and flow of your desires helps keep you from feeling overwhelmed by them and becomes as natural as putting on a sweater in response to coolness, and taking it off in response to warmth.

YOGA INQUIRY

Getting in Touch with the Body's Signals as Desires (GCFU)

This inquiry is divided into four stages, each getting progressively closer to discerning your body's signals. We'll do this process in downward-facing-dog pose — a pose that stretches the spine and legs. You will do the pose several times, so prepare yourself mentally for this repetition. I recommend that you read through the instructions first, and then take the book with you as you get down on the floor to do the exercise. This pose is best experienced on a non-slip surface, such as a yoga mat.

PART 1: NEUTRAL SENSATIONS

In the first round of the pose, you will start with the neutral sensations of the body.

1. Come down to the floor on all fours in table pose. Place your hands so they are shoulder width apart and your knees a few inches behind your hips.

2. Lift your hips and knees. Stretch back into downward-facing dog. Press firmly down with both hands and with strong arms. Dynamically reach your hips up and back. Breathe deeply into your belly. If you have short hamstrings and it is difficult to lengthen your spine, bend your knees.

3. Now, bring your attention to the "neutral" body sensations. Notice how the bones of your hands and toes make contact with the floor. Notice the texture of your yoga mat under your fingers and how the weight is distributed in your hands. Your mind will be prone to wandering. Fervency is your committed, deliberate attention directed toward this moment in your body, fired up against the urge for your mind to wander. Come back to the bones of your hands on the floor, your toes experiencing the texture of your

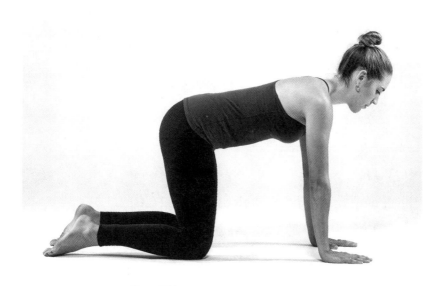

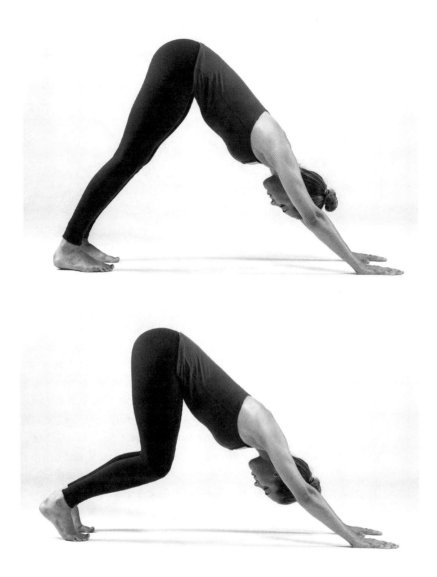

yoga mat. Notice these things with openness, with nonjudgmental curiosity. Limit yourself to taking in this specific information, even though your body will have many more sensations and your mind may be spinning with thoughts. Stay with this noticing for one minute.

4. Exhale and release into child's pose, a resting pose where your hips release back to your heels and your head and arms rest on the floor.

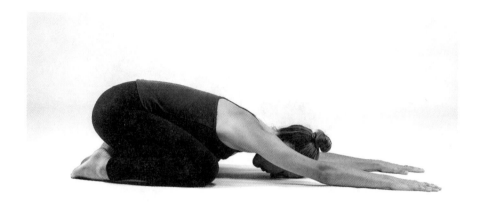

5. Acknowledge the fervency in your effort! Do not evaluate yourself. Fervency is your willingness to stick with the effort even if it feels awkward or confusing.

PART 2: NUANCED SENSATIONS

On the second round, we'll bring awareness to more nuanced sensations. Deliberately, keep this focus on your physical body, without entertaining any thoughts of judgment or evaluation about yourself. You may have the opportunity to notice how hard it is to suspend judgment! Fervency is your complete commitment to staying present to sensation. Because your mind will be prone to wander, this requires vigorous mental training. Fortunately, the body produces ever-fresh sensations for you to keep your mind engaged. Fervency is your commitment to this moment — and this moment — and this moment. Resist boredom, judgment, or feelings of foolishness.

1. Press back up into downward-facing-dog pose. Notice the strength required as you fully engage your arms to press your hands into your mat and to reach your hips away from your shoulders. Even more strongly awaken your arm muscles, like turning up the volume on the stereo. Notice how your arms and hips respond to this extra force.
2. Engage your leg muscles in a similar fashion, making them strong (but not locked; your knees are not meant to be locked). More strongly press your hips back toward the wall behind you and shift your weight into your legs. Notice again how your body responds to this increased effort. Feel the skin

of your body, the place between your shoulder blades, and even the way your eyes experience the pose. Limit what you notice to the experience in your body, without moving into story, critique, or judgments. Stay with this for one minute.

3. Exhale and release into child's pose.
4. Acknowledge the fervency in your effort! Do not evaluate yourself.

PART 3: BREATH SENSATIONS

On the third round, you'll create the same enthusiastic effort, but your attention will shift to the breath. This time your fervency will include complete commitment to the physical effort, without agitation or aggression, both of which would overwhelm your ability to connect with the breath.

1. Come into your downward dog with the enthusiasm of your "part 2" downward dog. Enliven your arms and legs, and deepen your breath into your lower abdomen.
2. While your muscles and bones continue to make strong effort, notice how your breath is moving. Consciously slow down your inhale and your exhale. Inhale and feel the breath moving into your body, the way a breeze wafts through the open window on a summer day. Patiently stay with your breath to the end of your exhale, the way that a breeze comes to stillness.
3. As you connect with your breath in this way, observe the effects. Quietly connect to any whisper of sensation inside. Does the lower abdomen feel more spacious, or more contracted? Is your breath smooth or choppy?
4. Stay connected to what you noticed, making notes in your mental journal. Stay with this for one minute.
5. Exhale and release into child's pose.
6. Acknowledge the fervency in your effort!

PART 4: DESIRE SENSATIONS

Finally, we'll do downward dog with the intention of exploring the sensations of desire. Before proceeding, rest a moment and scan your body, breath, and mind for what you're feeling. Specifically, investigate where you are on the spectrum of resistance or willingness, aversion or curiosity. I'll be blunt here and alert you to this: resistance and aversion will not move your recovery forward. Resistance and aversion are two of the main forces that swing the pendulum back and forth from desire to discipline.

1. At this juncture, fervency is your willingness to complete one more down-ward-facing-dog pose, on behalf of your recovery and your reawakened connection to your body's signals as messengers of desire. With this in mind, press up and back into downward-facing dog.
2. Does your body long to stretch more here or there? Are there other movements that your body craves?
3. As you stretch into downward dog, what does your heart rate do? Do you have a desire to breathe more deeply, more forcefully, more softly?
4. How does your stomach feel? Are there any identifiable signals of thirst, hunger, fullness or emptiness, heat or coolness? These might seem like basic questions to be asking yourself; don't dismiss them on these grounds. You need to get reacquainted with your body's signals. This is a part of the process.
5. Stay with your pose for one minute.
6. Exhale and release into child's pose.
7. Acknowledge the fervency in your effort!

Through these yoga practices, we invite body signals to be messengers of desire, knowing that all desire can be harnessed as an intelligent movement toward recovery. We can channel every small desire into our larger desire for awakening, ease, and resiliency. As we re-learn the language of body signals as desire, we will more quickly identify our urges to escape or numb out through old coping mechanisms. And we will know that those urges for escaping or numbing can be transformed into a deep desire for awakening. It is in the on-going process of tuning in to ourselves that we re-learn to trust the intelligence of life as it moves through us.

DISCIPLINE

On the other side of the pendulum from desire is discipline. The concept of discipline can be too easily exploited. When a compulsive or addictive behavior takes over our lives and prohibits us from experiencing even our most basic ease or capacity for happiness, we wonder why we have so little self-control, why we can't "get a handle on this." Usually these frustrations with ourselves are not accompanied by tenderness, genuine curiosity, or gentle-hearted sadness that could produce helpful responses. Rather, accompanying this confusion about our "lack of control" is profound self-loathing, despair, exasperation, or shame. When it comes to your body, you've probably had at least one of the following ideas about discipline, control, and self-acceptance:

- Once I reach a certain number on the scale, I'll be happy, satisfied, or acceptable (to myself or others).
- Hunger is something to be conquered.
- I should control my appetite.
- Feeling full is the same as feeling fat.
- Feeling full is also being numb. Numb is better than feeling.
- Feeling hungry is the same as feeling empty.
- Feeling empty is too uncomfortable.
- Feeling empty is sacred and safe.
- Cravings are dangerous.
- Intuitive eating will make me fat.
- If I give myself permission, I'll never stop eating.
- I must make it to the gym, run ten miles, or complete my exercise routine in order to be okay.
- I have to weigh myself every day (or many times a day). If I don't, I will lose control.
- If I eat that, I will have to purge it, take laxatives, or start burning calories right now.
- If I can make it through the day without eating anything, and have a small salad for dinner, then I will feel powerful, which is more important to me than feeling good, spontaneous, or free. I wouldn't know how to do those feelings anyway.
- Once I get control over all of this, I will love myself. I know I'm worth loving, somewhere underneath all of this.

Shortly, we'll look at what we are trying to get control over, how we trigger a biochemistry that makes us more vulnerable and less resilient (which makes what would otherwise be a matter of kind and simple self-discipline seem elusively out of reach), and what might be some of our most unhelpful messages about the nature of discipline itself. Because these discussions may challenge your current relationship to yourself, I encourage you to read slowly, patiently, and carefully. The discussions are potent, rich, and dense with important information. It will take time to digest these words. You may find you have to read sections more than once or that your eyes bounce off the page and your mind wanders. Some of this is the natural response of exposing your brain to a new language. Some of it may be a response of apprehension, as I will be asking you to shift the lens through which you see yourself. Please do your best to stick with me.

What we try to get "control over" is our behavior. Yet we are simultaneously waging war on ourselves, a war we cannot win through self-hatred. We hate our behaviors, and their accompanying thoughts and feelings. We hate ourselves for having them. Just like merging our "bad" behaviors with our "bad" desires, we merge our "bad" behaviors with our very "badness." As we try to manage this feeling of pervasive, internalized badness, otherwise known as shame, discipline comes to mean punishment, deprivation, retribution, and atonement. These attitudes reinforce our sense of "badness" and block us from the opportunity to learn about the root cause of our behavior. Without the ability to learn about why we're doing what we're doing, we're left with only our most unhelpful thinking: we do it because there is something terribly wrong with us. Painfully, this thought alone causes us to further contract around shame. The brain chemistry we create essentially programs us to live with the equivalent of an IV drip of anxiety and fear coursing through our body-mind-psyche. We're left with only our most basic protective (animal) instincts: fight, flight, freeze, or submit. Each of these becomes a very poor substitute for the foundation of discipline that could actually lead us out of the dense jungle of our mental patterns that initiate our addictive behaviors, reinforce shame, and keep us feeling helpless in the face of anxiety. Essentially, we've looped ourselves into a cyclical reinforcement of a no-win situation.

Reinforcing "Badness" and the Fight-Flight-Freeze-Submit Circuitry

Once we've reinforced our "badness" enough, it occurs as unconsciously as the reaction our hand has to a hot stove. We engage in "bad" behaviors and then experience ourselves as bad. An instinct arises to make up for this badness. We try to control our behavior or punish ourselves. To do this, we enact a rigorous plan for control of our behavior, a plan essentially flawed because it is steeped in self-loathing and causes us to disconnect from loving ourselves. Then control or punishment fails and we reengage with our "bad" behavior. We feel worse about ourselves and we know there is something terribly, terribly wrong with us. We experience ourselves as pervasively, intrinsically, irredeemably bad. We've reinforced shame by trying to use shame to overcome shame. As such, we've created an internal environment where we are constantly "under the influence" of shame, where we consistently run the programming for fight-flight-freeze-submit (FFFS).

With enough repetition through this cyclical reinforcement, it takes less and less to prompt its arousal and momentum. Sadly, we start to develop insidious and seductive mental strategies, disguised as discipline. For example, even a thought about how we will "discipline" or "motivate" ourselves for any badness — let's say a bite of brownie — temporarily ameliorates the pain of engaging in self-harming behavior again. The thought of how we will get ourselves under control, after this bite of brownie, also ameliorates our fear of this badness getting out of control. Essentially, we learn how to manipulate ourselves into permission for our "bad" behavior when we simultaneously plan our deprivation-control-discipline strategy and engage in our behaviors. We get caught in endless cycles of black-and-white thinking, acting and reacting, indulging and disciplining, "misbehaving" and "making up for."

Keep in mind that it is not the bite of brownie, or the numbers of bites of brownies, or even the brownies themselves that are the problem. Brownies are not bad. We are not bad for eating them. What's problematic is the thought process underneath all of this. Our dense jungle of mental patterns produces a biochemical, body-mind-psyche reaction when we see the brownie. We may even go through all four of the most basic animal instincts when we see the brownie:

Fight: fight with ourselves, or the brownie, about the temptation (preemptive self-scolding, decide on punishment strategy if indulging)

Flight: flee the scene, disconnect from our body, or hide the brownie in the cupboard (when under the influence of this brain spell, how long does that last?)

Freeze: tense up, clench teeth, get hypervigilant about the brownie, lose brain capacity for clear decision making about the brownie or, at times, other things, too

Submit: "oh, fuck it" . . . submit to the brownie, submit to badness taking over again

I know you may want to get control over the brownie, get some discipline over your behaviors. Yet our behaviors are symptoms, not causes. Of course, once in action, behaviors create more symptoms. Yoga suggests we address our symptoms at the root. To this end, I propose we head toward the root by working with our FFFS patterns.

BREATHING INTERVENTIONS: ANTIDOTES TO THE FFFS PATTERN

Although these are biologically programmed survival reactions, we have learned to trip ourselves into these reactions even when there is no real threat to our biological survival. We will also engage these reactions when we feel mentally, emotionally, or psychologically threatened. Shame and addiction set us up to feel threatened much more easily and frequently. Getting a handle on how to shift our mind-body reaction empowers us to reduce our vulnerability and increase our resilience.

FFFS patterns all have an associated breathing response in the body. To move to fight or flight, we trigger our secondary respiration muscles, those meant for an actual physical emergency that would require our ability to ward off or run fiercely away from a predator. Freeze or submit reactions shut down our breathing into miniscule sips of air, the tiniest amount of respiration needed — for example, in mimicking death (thus a predator might lose interest).

Yoga's antidotes to these reactions begin with shifting our breathing pattern back to diaphragmatic breathing. Diaphragmatic breathing is your body's natural resting breath. It is the breath of the relaxation response. It reduces anxiousness and calms the mind and body. Fortunately, the following breathing tools are completely accessible to any of us, any time.

Important note: If you practice on a daily basis, your body-mind circuitry will be better able to bring this on board as an antidote to the FFFS reaction. If you don't practice regularly, the techniques will still be potent, but they will require more fervency from you to remember the techniques, to do them, and to stick with them until the reaction dissolves and the antidotes work.

Fight Reaction Becomes Befriending

Befriending yourself in any circumstance is a powerful antidote to the habit of fighting with yourself. To warmly welcome your thoughts and feelings without reactivity or disappointment softens your nervous system, quiets your overactive resistant mind, and relaxes your physical body. To befriend your-self in a moment of anxious brownie craving does not mean that you eat the brownie. It means you radically accept and befriend your anxiety, your craving, and even your disappointment that, for now, a compulsively eaten brownie is not a choice you can make. In this process, you are becoming a better friend to yourself. Sensations, thoughts, and feelings will arise and pass. Each has a nuance and duration of its own. None of them is a permanent marker on your body or your mind. To befriend what is arising is to say *yes* to yourself, an espe-cially lifesaving skill when it comes to the most potent of feelings.

YOGA INQUIRY

Befriending Breathing Practice

1. Lie on your back with your knees bent.
2. Place your hands on your belly.
3. Welcome your chest to soften and welcome your breathing to relax into your belly. To welcome something to occur in a yoga exercise is to release any resistance that would block the invitation for your body to respond.
4. Notice any arising sensation or thought. As you inhale, extend a warm invi-tation to what is arising in your body or your mind.
5. As you exhale, further soften your chest and relax your belly, welcoming what is occurring for you into an inner space of warm acceptance.
6. Practice this for one to two minutes. Then rest and reflect for another minute.

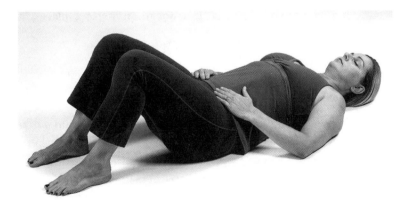

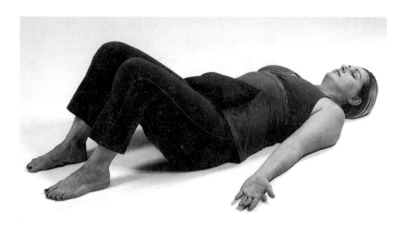

DEEPENING

This requires a ten-pound bag of sand or rice (a ten-pound bag of rice can be purchased at an international grocery store, such as an Asian store).

1. Place the ten-pound bag of rice on your abdomen. When you inhale, make an effort to push the rice bag up.
2. When you exhale, let the weight of the rice bag fall into your belly to support a more complete exhale. With this exhale, extend a warm welcome to yourself, and befriend whatever is arising as information and opportunity.

CHAIR VERSION

To practice discreetly in public, sit in a chair and place one hand on your lower belly. Bring your mind back to your reclined practice of befriending yourself, so as to awaken your mind-body memory and capacity. Then soften your breath into your belly. (If it is not too indiscreet, place your other hand on your heart; see next page.)

Flight Reaction Becomes Homecoming

Those of us who primarily move to the flight reaction under stress know well how to abandon ship, as it were. We have learned to flee the scene, leave behind important feelings and needs, and disengage from our body. Essentially, the flight reaction is a self-abandoning act. The following "homecoming" practice

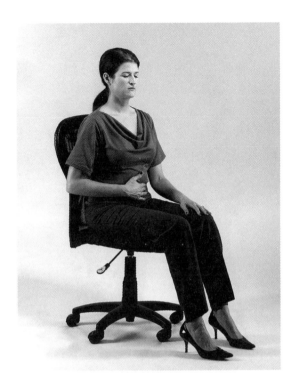

is our invitation, from ourselves and to ourselves, to come back home to our body, mind, feelings, needs, and desires.

YOGA INQUIRY

Homecoming Breathing Practice

1. Sitting in a chair (it doesn't matter whether or not the chair has arms), hook your arms over the back of the chair in a slightly slouched position or lightly hold your hands together at the small of your back. This disarms the secondary respiratory muscles of the upper chest.
2. Consciously invite yourself to return to your body, to drop into your breath, and to reconnect your mind to the tangible sensations of your body.
3. Notice your body's intelligence automatically knowing how to move into diaphragmatic breathing. Even without you having to choreograph this,

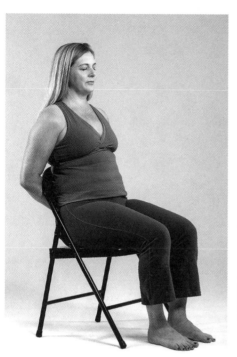

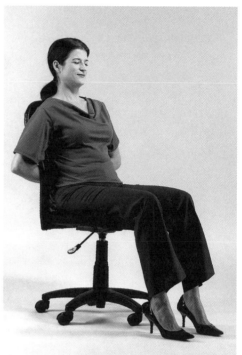

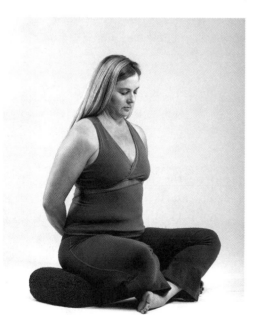

your body knows how to release the fight-flight breath and return to diaphragmatic breathing.

4. Mentally acknowledge your body's intelligent way of bringing you back home to yourself.

5. Your flight patterns have been strengthened by repetition. Acknowledge that this homecoming to ourselves can also be strengthened by repetition.

6. Practice this for one to two minutes. Then rest and reflect for another minute. (Note that this practice can also be done discreetly in public.)

SEATED MEDITATION VERSION

Sitting on a meditation cushion, lightly hold your hands together at the small of your back. Slightly tip your head forward.

Freeze Reaction Becomes Melting

The freeze reaction is intended to help us survive a threat that we either are unable or do not know how to fight off or flee from. Freezing acts a bit like frostbite, where all essential resources are redirected toward one thing: survival. In frostbite, this redirection is toward the core of the body to keep alive only what is essential, our internal organs. In the psychological freeze response, the body experiences heightened arousal and awareness of a perceived threat, while simultaneously becoming immobilized as all available resources are directed toward one thing: a decision about how to respond to the threat. Unfortunately, the way our nervous system becomes aroused creates a hypervigilant state in our body-mind-psyche, but not necessarily a fresh, intelligent response to the threat. With freeze as a survival reaction, we live in smaller and smaller circles of our life function, where we direct resources toward scanning the environment for cues, rather than exploring our world for its creativity, mystery, and majesty. We also freeze emotions that we are unable to experience, like when something gets frozen in winter ice. Melting is the delicate art of thawing from within. Akin to releasing tension from the body or mind, melting occurs as we mentally invite an area of holding to let go. We may have experienced similar letting go if we've had a massage or taken a hot bath, which are both invitations from the outside in. Melting is an invitation from the inside out.

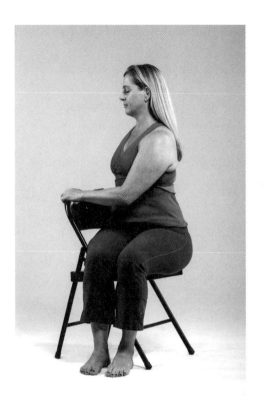 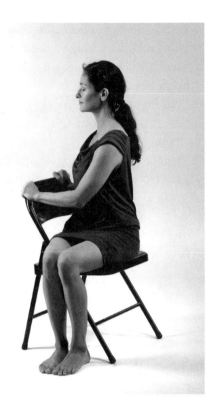

❧ YOGA INQUIRY

Melting Breathing Practice

1. Take a seat in a chair — one without arms, if possible.
2. Turn to your right and sit sideways on the chair.
3. Twist your upper body to the right. Hold the back of the chair with each hand. Use your hands to support you in twisting gently. This does not need to be vigorous for it to work.
4. Now bring your attention to your belly and your breath.
5. With each exhale, allow any tension in your body or mind to melt.
6. Soften the skin of your body and let your shoulder blades melt down your back.

7. Soften the skin between your eyebrows and relax the hinge of your jaw.
8. Most important, welcome this melting to start thawing any holding, tightness, or tension in your belly. When your eyes soften, soften your belly. When you relax your tongue, relax your mind.
9. Welcome the belly to melt its holding patterns, knowing that you are softening to yourself. For these moments, there is no predator and you are not in danger. You do not need to freeze up or contract.
10. Practice this for one to two minutes on each side. Then rest and reflect for another minute.

Melting takes time. It will only happen incrementally, which is a healthy process, much like thawing frostbite. With frostbite, we don't plunge the affected limb into hot water. We don't even use warm water. In initiating the process of thawing frostbite, the water temperature is cool, so as to invite the body to recirculate blood into the affected area slowly. This process causes less damage and is medically recommended. In the same manner, your body's approach to melting will be incremental. Practice this breathing daily, lovingly, and you will experience the melting at a pace that your body can tolerate.

Submit Reaction Becomes Inflating

The submit reaction is much like a possum playing dead. In submit as a survival reaction, we become resigned and experience a profound loss of hope. In response to the perceived threat, we give up our capacity to confront (fight), our wherewithal to flee (flight), and our vigilant scanning for options (freeze). Psychologically, we may experience states of numbness and apathy. We may feel time dramatically slowing down, experience a dismissive response to pain, or have the sense of "seeing ourselves as if from across the room." Physiologically, our body withdraws all resources away from fight, flight, or freeze, and greatly reduces how much resource is even "online." Our autonomic nervous system responds with lowered heart rate, lowered blood pressure, and shallow to almost nonexistent breathing. Inflating is like when we blow up a balloon or inflate a bicycle tire. While our aim is to inflate the lungs, we're also energetically inflating our courage and commitment too.

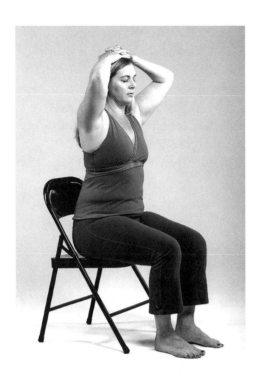 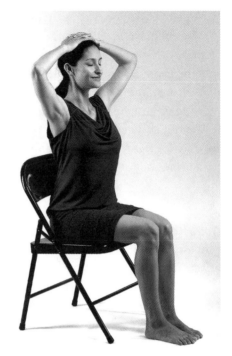

⤳ YOGA INQUIRY

Inflating Breath Practice

1. Sit comfortably in a chair or on the floor.
2. Clasp your hands and rest them on top of your head. Positioning your arms in this manner prevents your body from using secondary respiration muscles and opens your thoraco-abdominal cavity for deeper breathing.
3. With your hands resting on top of your head, bring your attention down into your physical body. Inhabit your muscles and bones, and connect with the chair or floor on which you are sitting.
4. Feel the density of your physical contact with the environment beneath you.
5. Welcome your breath to deepen slightly, within your comfort zone.
6. You might imagine this like inflating a balloon inside your torso. With each inhale, slowly expand that balloon to touch your abdomen, ribs, and back waist from the inside.

7. With each exhale, soften your efforts so as to rest into, rather than over-whelm, yourself.

8. Practice this for one to two minutes. Then rest and reflect for another minute.

This can be done discreetly in public. In fact, we've all seen people lean-ing back in a chair or sitting on a park bench with their hands resting on top of their head. We may also have seen someone deep in reflective thought sitting similarly at their desk, reclined back, legs crossed, hands on top of the head.

FFFS and the Cycle of Shame

Here's the juice: your "inability" to discipline yourself is rooted in shame, cat-alyzed by underlying and repeated biochemical flushes of FFFS, sustained by neurologically grooved habit, and filled with significant power that you could instead use to liberate yourself.

Let's look at a simple analogy. When we put our hand on the hot stove, the circuitry that runs through us to promptly lift our hand away from danger doesn't require our rational, reasoning, thinking mind. We're neurologically and physiologically programmed for our hand to whisk itself off of the hot stove without having to learn it, remember it, or practice it. It's a self-protective mechanism, a lifesaving instinct.

Shame, the experience of feeling we are deeply flawed, inadequate, or irre-deemably bad, is to our addiction what the hot stove is to our hand. Shame is a threat to our survival. In creating our survival strategies, we were attempting to defend ourselves against the shame we were exposed to in our environ-ment, directly or indirectly. When we internalized shame — that is, when we took over the shame messages broadcast from our environment and began broadcasting them to ourselves — we changed our programming, such that it became necessary to defend against our own shame broadcast, against our very being. From the inside, we trigger and retrigger our own shame threats, most often in the form of a condescending, overbearing, self-critical voice that regularly narrates negative self-judgments. We trigger our FFFS reaction and fuel ourselves to be on guard against shame, both from within ourselves and from our environment. Shame is the hot stove of our emotional mind. It doesn't get processed through our rational mind. In a blink, shame whisks us into FFFS patterns to defend ourselves. Every time we engage with shame in this way, we are circulating this through our body-mind-psyche, increasing our vulnerability, decreasing our resilience, and greatly reducing the likelihood that we will be able to "discipline" ourselves from our wise mind. For recovery, we will use the yoga tool discussed earlier, of moving from love, not shame, to intervene on shame's efforts to discipline us with punishment or condemnation.

Moving from Love, not Shame: Nonpunishing,
Nonshaming Attitude (MLNS)

Having sensations, body signals, desires, or "lack of discipline" is not the result of you having done something wrong, and you do not need to be punished. Besides which, punishing, or shaming, yourself (1) doesn't make the sensations better; (2) doesn't let you learn anything new; (3) increases the likelihood of the same sensations, body signals, or desires returning, only stronger; and (4) adds to the biochemical rush that will produce additional sensations, body signals, and desires that overwhelm your ability to cultivate helpful discipline strategies. Using a self-punishing approach is actually a great way to stay stuck, ensuring that what you're now experiencing will become cyclical.

Nonpunitive care sounds like a mouthful. Nonshaming? Another mouthful. Yet I want to make this point really clearly. Moving from love is the *absence* of punishing or shaming ourselves. A yogic approach uses words in an interesting way when talking about specific attitudes. Take, for example, the teachings on *ahimsa*. *Himsa* means "violence." The letter *a* translates as "the absence of." So *ahimsa* is the "absence of violence," or nonviolence. It wasn't written as compassion, or kindness, or niceness. It was very specifically written as the absence of violence — that is, nonviolence.

In this same regard, even though I'm asking for a mouthful from you, consider that nonpunishing or nonshaming is actually inherently more powerful for your mind to register than gentleness or kindness is. Don't get me wrong — there's a place for these qualities, too. But when it comes to learning to be gentle or kind to ourselves, that can sound a little too wimpy, and it doesn't get to the deeper pain of the matter. We've been punishing and shaming ourselves. And that hasn't worked! Now, we are going to be nonpunishing and nonshaming. Learning to feel the effect of punitive, shaming self-talk is one way to make this shift.

YOGA INQUIRY

Explore a Nonshaming Attitude (MLNS)

Let yourself become still and quiet. Relax your face, your jaw, and your breathing. Become aware of the temperature in the room and any peripheral noises. Then bring your attention to your thoughts. When you're ready, spend a minute on each of the following questions:

- How do I think when I am punishing or shaming myself? Clearly? Calmly? With a scolding tone? With a loving tone? Angrily? Anxiously? With a sense of deflation? With despair? With motivation?
- How does my body respond to this thinking? What happens with my heart rate, breath rate, or body temperature?
- What could be hopeful about nonpunishing or nonshaming thinking?
- What feels scary about using a nonpunishing attitude with myself?
- How does my body respond to these possibilities?
- How does my body respond when I consider:

    a voice tone of self-kindness?

    a moment of self-appreciation (for my strength, willingness, earnestness)?

    words of self-respect?

    statements of real appreciation for myself?

This inquiry is meant to stimulate your intuition through your body's intelligence. Disordered eating, addiction, and self-harming behaviors bury this intelligence, and we now want to unearth it and hold it close.

Is It Shame or Intelligence?

Yoga uses the term *intelligence* to refer to an overarching, innately wise, physiologically embedded mind-body movement toward growth. We can think of this intelligence in two ways. One is to see it as the profound and magical complexity of our physical body, including all of its known and unknown functions, its ability to constantly adapt to its inner and outer environment, such as fluctuating temperatures, and its capacity to integrate adaptations as our species evolves. A second way to see this is as a magnetic pull from life itself for us to grow — to grow in capacity, competency, and vitality — in our mind, body, and heart.

We have the power to influence each of these intelligences. We can learn to follow the innate wisdom of our body-mind, or we can ignore, interrupt, or mistrust this wisdom. When we do the latter, we experience the friction of this disconnect as symptoms, such as anxiety, depression, or addiction. But what if your addiction was this overarching intelligence trying to get your attention to bring you back on course? What if the symptoms of your "lack of discipline" were important messages from your body-mind intelligence?

❧ YOGA INQUIRY

Shame or Intelligence? (MLNS)

Again, let yourself become still and quiet. Relax your face, your jaw, and your breathing. Become aware of the temperature in the room and any peripheral noises. Then bring your attention to your thoughts. When you're ready, spend a minute on each of these reflections as messages your body may be trying to send you, through the medium of your addiction, shame, and rebellion. With each message, notice how your body responds. Observe your heart rate, breath rate, restlessness, or curiosity.

- *Your addiction has been a self-protective mechanism all along.* You've been circulating shame, in the form of thought (and resulting behavior), through your body-mind-psyche for years, causing yourself to whisk into compulsive, self-protective strategies.
- *Shame causes you to rebel against yourself.* Disciplining yourself with shame will produce a self-protective strategy in the form of rebellion. Thus, you rebel against your own plans of action!
- *This rebellion is a sign of your deepest urge for freedom from shame.* When you rebel, even with the self-harming behaviors of your addiction, the strength of that rebellion is a measure of the strength of your desire to be free. However, you're behaving in ways that are also painful and undermining your ability to find freedom. The act of rebellion is in itself intelligent because it attempts to ward off the self-induced pain of the punitive, shame-based discipline. (Like the hand being whisked off the stove.)
- *The "plan maker" in you reveals your potential to actualize this freedom.* Although your "plan maker" is often perfectionistic, demanding, overly rigid,

and unrealistic, the fact that the plan maker is still active in your system is a sign of your potent, healthy drive toward capacity and freedom.

The more time you spend in shame-based discipline, arousing the biochemistry of your FFFS system, the more vulnerable you are to shame, simply because the FFFS system increases the vulnerability of your entire system. In a near-constant state of arousal of our FFFS pattern, we will experience pervasive restlessness, a restlessness that looks for an outlet to soothe it. Food! Ah-ha! We learned that food does this so well! In fact, it too has a biochemical impact on our body-mind. Food can be used as medicine. Yet we've been using food to self-medicate. Things like caffeine, sugar, carbohydrates, fat, salt, stimulants, and alcohol do shift our physiology, and, in some cases, this is the only relief we've known how to create. Exercising and restricting food also have biochemical impacts on our FFFS system. They, too, can be medicinal, as in proper exercise, and proper fasting, cutting back or cleaning up our diet. Yet, again, they can also be used to self-medicate. When we're self-medicating with food, exercise, or restriction, we're interrupting our body's ability to intelligently self-regulate.

The more time you spend practicing the reduction of your FFFS pattern, the greater control you will have over it. Practicing, even when you are not triggered — in fact, especially when you are not triggered — is profoundly important. You are essentially building up the antibodies for when your body needs them most. Similar to building up your immune system before flu season, you'll be less vulnerable and, when you do get triggered, your body will be more deeply programmed to respond with resilience rather than helplessness. The more time you spend recognizing shame as an invasive mind-body virus, something separate from you, and something incapable of defining you, the freer you will be from its power.

Likewise, the more time you spend acknowledging your victories over this cycle, even the smallest of wins, the stronger you'll feel about continuing on. You'll build your faith in yourself and in your new process for discipline, or what you may come to call fervency.

Shaking Off Your FFFS

Our personal FFFS pattern has been ingrained through repetition since we were very young. Our body knows precisely how to respond to our mental perceptions of the world around or within us. When our mind is sparked into our FFFS pattern, without an additional ounce of attention, focus, or input from us, our body tightens the chest, sends a hot flash of sensation, and restlessly engages in self-soothing behaviors. We're experiencing these things because something has frightened us. We've registered a threat in our environment.

Once the FFFS system is triggered, our body will look for an outlet. For example, animals in the wild, and even my little dog at home, will automatically "shake off" their body's FFFS reaction, once the threat is over. Almost daily I observe my dog get caught up in some kind of anxiousness. I can practically see his brain running a movie in his head. He has very specific ways of barking, moving, and then releasing the stress. Two of his favorite options include vigorously shaking his head, left-right-left-right, ears flapping to make helicopter noises, until he feels settled; and running up to one of his stuffed animal chew toys, grabbing it in his mouth, and shaking it side to side while growling at it. He does this instantly and for a short burst. Again, he does this until he has settled his FFFS reaction. At that moment, I can literally see he has transformed himself out of his FFFS spell. He's done this without leaving any residue.

We, too, need outlets for the biochemistry of our FFFS reactions. Yet, most often, we don't intelligently tend to ourselves. We've blocked our body's ability to give us clear signals about what to do, and we've blocked our ability to hear even the faint signals of body intelligence that could tell us. Consider the following experience, for example.

You're driving on the freeway going just above the speed limit, but not much above the flow of traffic. In your rearview mirror, you see police lights. You quickly check your own speed and the car next to you. You can't be sure whether the police car is after you or not, but your mind-body system has already flushed to alert. You might feel your heart rate increase, your mouth get dry, your stomach flutter, your hands grip the wheel, your mind make flash suggestions ("step on the brake, don't step on the brake, act calm and cool"), or all of the above. In another moment, the police car has gone by you. It wasn't after you. Whew!

You recognize you're not getting pulled over. A wave of relief comes over you. Yet, even though you know you are not under immediate threat, your body doesn't make an immediate shift out of the FFFS reaction. It takes time for this to settle down (physiologically about twenty minutes). You might find yourself taking a deeper breath, which your body signaled to help you calm

⚬ *Flight-Fight-Freeze-Submit (FFFS) Accumulation*

We register a perceived threat in our environment (internal or external). It may include the threat of judgment, abandonment, rejection, exposure, or annihilation. To ward off the threat, our FFFS system revs up. This both floods the body with the biochemistry of FFFS and shuts down vital resources. (Under threat the body suppresses digestive, endocrine, and immune function.) After a threat, the body must come down from the surge and overcome the suppression of those vital resources. Yet when we self-medicate, attempting to soothe our pain, it blocks the body's ability to come down or to overcome the suppression.

We then acclimate to higher FFFS biochemistry. This lowers our threshold for new threats (stress, and so forth), causes fatigue, increases our vulnerability, decreases our resilience, and narrows our life bandwidth. It also sets us up for health challenges (anxiety, pain, depression, heart disease, diabetes, chronic pain, and the like).

down. You might find yourself brushing your hair off your face, reaching for a sip of water, or opening the window for fresh air. Your body has signaled these actions, too.

If you've buried your body's signals, however, you may not get these messages. It will take longer for your system to come down from the event. You may find yourself with a food craving or an urge to engage in harmful behaviors. These efforts to self-medicate, to "bring you down" from the FFFS-triggering event, will further trigger your body with the biochemical storm of compulsive food behaviors, including the accompanying mental storms of regret, self-loathing, and urges for punitive discipline. Sadly, in contrast to my little dog's technique, these self-medicating strategies are not "residue-free." We don't get to resolve the FFFS reaction from the triggering event, because we interrupted our body's natural ability to do so. Not only do we keep a layer of the original FFFS reaction circulating, but we've also added a layer of self-medicated body chemistry and, in response to that, a layer of shame in the form of self-loathing and punishment.

When we aren't able to identify, respond to, and resolve these episodes of FFFS reactions, our body learns to acclimate to living with accumulated levels of this biochemistry circulating all the time. With this, we're much more susceptible to triggers from the inner or outer environment; it takes much less for us to become triggered, and when we do get triggered, we have less room left for our body's intelligent response. We've programmed ourselves to be more vulnerable and less resilient. Both of these neurobiological states make what would otherwise be wise and skillful discipline difficult to grasp because our animal body will already be prepared for defensive or offensive maneuvers against incoming "threats."

BREATHING INTERVENTIONS: SHAKING OFF FFFS

Just about any movement process can help you shift your physiology out of the FFFS reaction. Here are some specific practices to help when you've been triggered. Keep in mind that the breathing practices to support you in befriending, homecoming, melting, and inflating are still critical daily tools for you to create a physiological shift that will build your body-mind resilience. That shift promotes changes in your endocrine, digestive, and immune systems, all of which are taken offline during an emergency. (Essentially, during an emergency our body does not need to consider reproducing offspring, digesting whatever is in our stomach, or fighting off the flu.) Therefore, it's important to keep this in mind when we do experience a triggering event, even if we are the cause of it, like looking in the mirror and falling into a pit of self-hatred. Every time we experience a trigger, our body will follow its base programming to redirect resources to reacting to the threat. When we don't shake off the incident, our endocrine, digestive, and immune functions continue to be influenced, often operating at a suboptimal level.

⤶ SLUG SHAKING (PB)

1. Stand with your feet a bit wider than hip distance. Imagine you have something very sticky on your left hand and you need to vigorously shake it off. (In the Pacific Northwest we can imagine shaking off the slime of a slug. Yuck!)
2. Shake your left hand and arm vigorously. Move through forward, back, side, and overhead positions. Shake it for one minute without stopping.

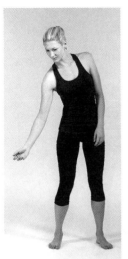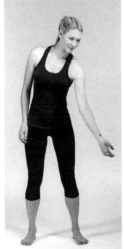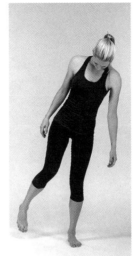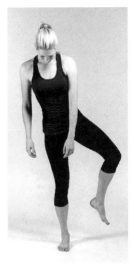

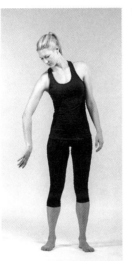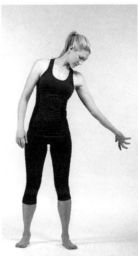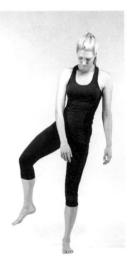

3. Repeat with your right arm.
4. Repeat with your left leg.
5. Repeat with your right leg.
6. Now stand perfectly still and notice what is occurring in your body.
7. Inhale deeply through both nostrils. Pause slightly and then exhale completely. Repeat this breath three times.

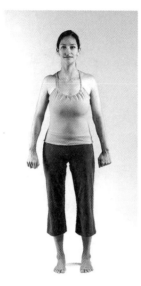
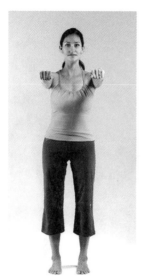
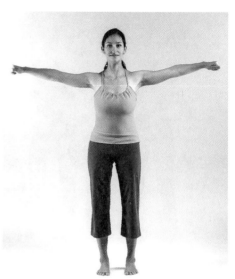
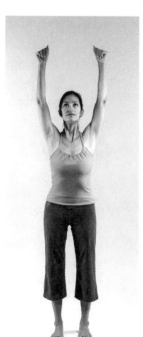
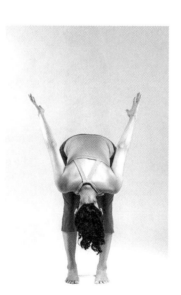

BREATH OF JOY (PB)

1. Stand with your feet a bit wider than hip distance. Bend your knees slightly and root your tailbone, somewhat like sitting on a horse.
2. With your hands as fists you're going to swing your arms into three different positions while inhaling briskly three times. (You could imagine this like how a cheerleader would swing her pom-poms.)
3. Inhale, swing arms forward.
4. Inhale, swing arms sideways.
5. Inhale, swing arms up overhead.
6. Exhale completely by sighing out your mouth (make some noise! growl if you need to!) while quickly folding forward and swinging your arms down past your legs. Open your hands as the exhale finishes, to further shake off anything that blocks your joy.
7. Do eight rounds.
8. At the end of eight rounds, hang down in the forward bend for a few moments and notice what your body is experiencing.
9. Stand up, inhale deeply through both nostrils, pause slightly, and then exhale completely. Do this three times.

PRESSURE-RELEASE-VALVE BREATHING (PB)

This practice can be done standing or sitting. It is intended to deliberately increase the intra-abdominal pressure as a way to bring on a more profound release of body-based, FFFS tension.

1. Place your hands on your head, as in the inflating breath practice.
2. Inhale slowly and deeply through your nose. Do your best to get a full-body breath (see next page, top left photo).
3. At the top of your inhale, hold the breath in. To make this more doable, snug your lower belly in a bit and drop your chin slightly. This seals the breath in the chamber of the torso (see next page, top right photo).
4. Before you exhale, release the seal (like taking the lid off of a jar), then exhale slowly through your mouth with pursed lips while simultaneously and slowly lowering your arms. Make the exhale longer than the inhale.

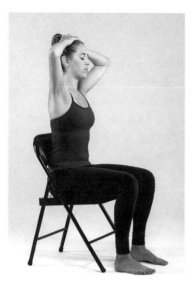
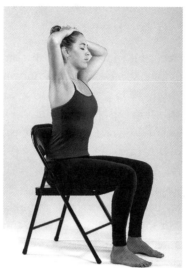
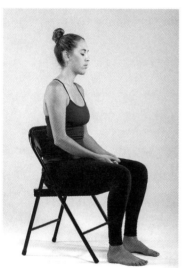

5. Pause for a quiet moment while your body takes a few smaller breaths.
6. Do this sequence three times.
7. Now repeat the sequence three times without your hands on your head.
8. At the end, sit quietly and notice any changes in your mind, body, and breath.

Yoga's Paradigm Shift for Discipline: Self-Nurturing Discipline

Through yoga, there is an entirely fresh relationship to discipline available to you. Self-nurturing discipline is a balanced blend of qualities that will transform your relationship to what has thus far been self-punitive discipline steeped in shame. Self-nurturing discipline is the process of (1) mindful attention; (2) acknowledging what is just for this moment; (3) nonpunitive, nonshaming attitude; (4) whole-brain discipline skills; and (5) reasonable guidelines that respect your body's innate intelligence and that nurture your life vitality. We've already explored numbers 1, 2, and 3. Now let's look at numbers 4 and 5.

WHOLE-BRAIN DISCIPLINE

The early stages of recovery will require consistent fervency on your part. For this to work, your brain is going to need to be convinced of an approach to discipline that is agreeable enough to motivate you and effective enough to yield results. The logical part of your brain (left hemisphere) will want a discipline that is scientific: definable, linear, and measurable. "Eat this. Don't eat that. Do this. Don't do that." Although I do recommend a discipline that is scientific, it will not work if it is dehumanized through black-and-white thinking, rigid control strategies, shame, or self-punishment. It will not work if you continue to treat yourself in alienating ways. You've already run those experiments. And I've seen them run with countless women, all with the same outcome: lowered self-esteem, increased levels of stress hormones, bigger backlashes in their disordered eating behavior, increased anxiety, and decreased faith in themselves.

The "other" (right hemisphere) part of your brain will want a discipline that saves you, forever, from the underlying pain pathways that have created the cyclical behavior patterns that lead to despair, helplessness, and confusion. This part of your brain will want a discipline that intuitively and kindly brings you back home to a you that is radiant, clear, confident, and expansive. This part of your brain will not want to be boxed into a linear protocol for the "rest of your life" (notice the power of this kind of overused language). Yet the logical part of your brain will not be comfortable being completely open-ended and intuitive for the "rest of your life."

Recovery through fervency is forged by a healthy interweaving of these two very alive frictions of the human spirit. On the one hand, we want control, logic, or reason. On the other hand, we want freedom and spontaneity!

Whole-brain discipline means applying the strengths of each hemisphere of our brain consistently. To do so, we start with a third force that our ancient yogis knew fundamentally: wise humility.

Discipline as Wise Humility

Within the word *discipline* is the concept of discipleship: a humble, dedicated, selfless attention to an art form (e.g., music), a practice (e.g., yoga), or any opportunity for development, as when someone becomes an apprentice to a master in a craft, or a student of a teacher in a particular tradition. To be a disciple of something is to offer oneself to it. In this, we recognize we can't already know what we still have to learn. We become learners. We become humble. Many, many times women have expressed these nearly universal frustrations:

- I already *know* what I should be doing, but I'm not doing it! What is wrong with me?
- Why don't I already know how to do this? I don't know how to feed myself, or let myself rest when I need to. What's the matter with me?
- How come I didn't learn this a long time ago?

None of those frustrations will put us in the optimal brain state for learning, nor do they let us explore wise humility and good studentship. Wise humility lets us say, "We're okay not already knowing." When we're willing to not know, we have room in our brain for learning something new. This is illustrated by stories of meditation masters who keep pouring tea into an already full mug; the student sees the tea running over the sides and shouts for the teacher to stop pouring. Yet he does not stop. He is illustrating that a full mug cannot take in any more tea. Likewise, a mind that is too full of what it thinks it knows can't take in new information.

One way to define discipline as wise humility is that we become a "disciple" of our body's innate intelligence and majesty. We've spent much time ignoring, mistrusting, and overriding this intelligence, and we've seen the outcomes of that. Yoga is truly an invitation for discipleship to the incredible intelligence of nature, as it lovingly cares for us. For each of us, it is an invitation to return to a respectful, humble, and committed relationship to your body. I know this might sound tremendously unappealing right now. It might even sound ridiculous.

"If she only knew how messed up my body is!" I know this thought. I heard it in my own head. I've heard it from countless women. I've also seen miracles, in the span of five minutes. I've witnessed women coming back to humility and discipleship to their body's intelligence. And I've seen their bodies respond!

"Trust my body's intelligence? What is that?!" It is the intelligence that beats your heart, breathes your lungs, regulates your body temperature, and alerts you to the sensations, signals, and symptoms of your body being in alignment, or out of alignment, with its own intelligence.

"Listening to my body is what got me into this mess in the first place!" Truly, deeply, respectfully listening to your body cannot create a mess. However, your body might be experiencing a "mess" of internal efforts to keep up with or overcome the damages you've done.

In the process of learning any new art form, wise humility teaches us to start with three key elements: attention to the basics, repetition of the new skills, and a willingness to be a learner, not an already accomplished artisan. When I learned to play the trumpet, for example, I had to learn how to hold the instrument, how to position my mouth on the mouthpiece, and how to breathe properly to make sound come out. I learned the combination of fingerings to create countless musical notes. And I practiced scales over and over again, up and down, up and down. Finally, I had to be able to hear the sounds coming from my trumpet. I was taught to listen and, through listening, I learned to identify when I was playing sharp, flat, too loud, too soft, too fast, or too slow.

The music came alive after my new skills were developed through repetition, and when, through humility (afforded to me by a combination of my personal insecurity as a musician and my awe that composers wrote such beautiful music), I learned to let the music come through me. Likewise, in the process of yoga, when we start with the basics, practice repetition, and learn to listen, we will grow into an immeasurable artistry with ourselves. We will experience life coming through us like music through an instrument. We will learn the new skill of truly listening to ourselves.

Fervency: Humility + Repetition = New Skill

When we learn a new skill, we fire new neural pathways in our brain. One of the definitions of fervency is constancy in an effort toward a goal. The efforts you apply to your recovery, repeated day after day, will become skills: yoga skills, recovery skills, and life skills. Discussing the "sound panel" metaphor

(p. 36), I used the term *survival skill* to describe disordered eating behavior. Essentially, through specific experiences, external and internal, you picked up a learned behavior that was soothing in some way (even if it was also painful or confusing) and repeated it again and again. It was helpful to you. It became a survival skill, a self-soothing skill. It also became self-harming. Keep in mind as you develop the until-now-missing life skills that yoga teaches, you will want to employ repetition and constancy to embed them into your brain to become a more powerful go-to resource than your old skill was.

The skill of disordered eating behavior does not grow with you; in fact, it prevents you from growing and evolving psychologically and spiritually. But the skills of yoga grow and evolve over time, when practiced with humility and repetition. Learning to regulate your breathing with a technique called *ujjayi* is one yoga skill that can become a way to regulate your mind and gain some control over your FFFS patterns.

❧ FERVENCY BREATHING TOOLS

Humilty + Repetition = New Skills

Ujjayi Breath

Ujjayi translates as "victorious breath." Think of this as "victory over" your unhelpful mental habits, your shame broadcasts, your restlessness, distractedness, or uneasiness. I like to think of it as our Jedi Knight breath, from *Star Wars*. May the force be with you! To "tap into" the force, as it were, practice the ujjayi breath technique.

1. Place the tip of your tongue behind your top two teeth. Open the back of the throat and make it hollow. As your draw the breath in and out, the air will pass through your nose, but you will feel your body drawing the breath more through the hollow of your throat. Nose breathing, without the ujjayi technique, can sound like a long sniff or sigh. This is not what we are going for here, and it does not have the same effect on your mind. Throat breathing, as I'll call it sometimes, has a distinct whispering quality to it that is even and smooth on both the inhale and the exhale. The contraction of the epiglottis in the back of the throat creates this sound. It is the same contraction you would use to whisper or that happens when you yawn. If you have trouble creating the ujjayi sound, try exhaling through

your mouth using a whispering sound or yawn deliberately and notice the shape at the back of your throat. Use that same shape to inhale and exhale through your nose.

2. The throat creates the structure, as does your mental focus and the time you dedicate. Repetition of this breathing technique will help it become more familiar and more powerful very quickly.

3. For this introduction to ujjayi breathing, try practicing the breath, with its sound and smoothness, for two uninterrupted minutes. Close the book and close your eyes. Make a deliberate effort to do nothing other than this breath. Focus your entire listening and your mental attention on the sound and movement of the breath in the back of your throat. Do nothing else. This is the breath of victory. As such, concentrate and cultivate the force of your conviction for recovery, for victory over shame.

4. At the end of two minutes, sit still without any effort applied to the breath. Simply remain quiet and observe the effects of the ujjayi breath.

UPWARD HANDS BREATH

In the following exercise, we'll be using the ujjayi breath and the upward movements of your arms in tandem, choreographed by the long, slow pace of your breath.

1. Stand tall (or sit tall in a chair). Join your palms together at your heart in a gesture called *Anjali mudra.*

2. As you inhale, sweep your arms out to the sides and up overhead. Fill your lungs from bottom to top, like how you would fill a glass of water. To do this, imagine filling the lower belly first (even though your lungs don't go that far down in your trunk, it helps to think of it this way), then fill the midtorso, and then your heart and upper chest. Move your arms in rhythm with this filling: the arms are lower when filling the lower belly, stretch out to the side as the midtorso gets inflated, then reach up overhead as the breath reaches the top of the inhale. Be deliberate about matching these movements to your breath. Finish the overhead reach as your inhale finishes.

3. Exhale, move your arms slowly to match the length of your breath cycle, moving them in the reverse order. Finish with joining your palms as your exhale finishes.

4. Inhale and repeat. Make the pace and timing slow and deliberate. Bring your entire attention to the concert of movement choreographed by your breath pace.

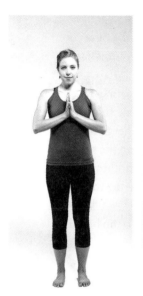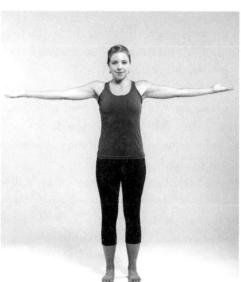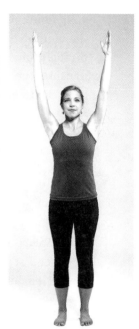

5. With your inhale, connect to the strength of your will to recover. With your exhale, forcibly say *no* to shame.
6. At a minimum, do this five times. For longer practice, do this for three minutes.
7. When you complete the last exhale, rest your hands in your lap (if sitting) or your arms by your sides (if standing), and relax in simple awareness.

As you're learning both of these breathing practices, I want you to honor the structure of how to perform the ujjayi breath and, in the upward hands breathing practice, the instruction to pace your arms with your breath. In the second exercise it is essential that you practice being led by your breath pace. This is one of the ways that yoga teaches us humility: let the breath be the conductor of the orchestra of muscles and bones. If you don't watch this carefully, I guarantee your mind will step in and start trying to pace this exercise for you. Most likely, it will want your arms to lead and for your breath to follow. This will keep you in the part of your brain that wants control. And in this exercise, that isn't worth reinforcing. Here we let the breath be the guide. Your arms surrender to the pace of your inhale and exhale. Your mind surrenders to the movements of the body. As I tell my students: be in the audience of the breath. Witness, appreciate, and respect this. It is teaching you good studentship and wise humility. Through wise humility you will discover a relationship to the breath that is breathing you (which it is doing right now), and to the energy of life that is sustaining you — the same vitality that causes flowers to come into bloom and compels birds to sing.

Repeating these practices day after day will teach you the skills of paying attention, pacing your breath and body in harmony, slowing down your mind, and fueling your fervency for recovery. By ritualizing these practices as the tools of wise humility, you embed them with meaning. Then, when shame arises and you feel the urge to condemn yourself with rigid control strategies or abandon your self-respect into chaotic behaviors, you can come directly back to this wise humility practice to reorient yourself and your relationship to self-nurturing, not self-punitive, discipline.

Discipline as Science

With a foundation of wise humility, we can now engage your desire for a linear, scientific, regulated discipline. Scientists observe, study, and respond objectively to the experiments they run. To do so, they must be objective, clear, humble, and open-minded (wise humility!). Simultaneously, they can bring great passion and intuition to their work.

Similarly, as we undertake the practices of yoga, a certain amount of scientific objectivity toward ourselves combined with respect for the tools necessary to benefit from yoga will support us in realizing more powerful discoveries. As someone with disordered eating patterns, you've already run countless body-based experiments that, in fact, have led to discoveries:

- Bingeing at night affects your sleep.
- Overeating impacts your weight.
- Chronic restricting impairs your brain function.
- Overexercising, or purging through exercise, is time-consuming and exhausting.
- Compulsive behaviors are profoundly painful and cause despair.

But those experiments were run blindly, impulsively, robotically. They were not run scientifically. Nor did they challenge the repeated outcomes for different results using new behaviors. Those experiments didn't include *fervency* as a scientific demand. Now they will.

FERVENCY: STRUCTURE + HEAT = TRANSFORMATION

Here is a household example of a science experiment to help us understand this equation. When you fill a teapot with water, you are containing the water within the structure of the teapot. When you set it on the stove, you have positioned the teapot for a potential transformation of the water. When you light the stove and establish the proper amount of flame, you will heat the teapot, thus heating the water inside. That fire transforms the water into steam. And when the water is securely held within the teapot and proper heat is applied, it will be helpless to become anything other than steam.

However, the experiment will fail if (1) the teapot has holes in it, (2) the teapot is not positioned on the stove, or (3) no one turns the heat on. It's important to realize an additional element about the heat: the water will eventually be transformed even with the smallest amount of fire, but it will take much more time for the transformation to happen, a duration in which you might get distracted, forgetful, impatient, or bored.

Likewise, when you arrange your recovery with healthy structure and apply the proper amount of heat (fervency in the form of consistent self-nurturing discipline), you will be helpless to do anything other than transform yourself. From a yoga perspective, the proper structure will include things like the time and location for your yoga practice (such as a class you might take or a place in your home in which you practice) and the nonnegotiable commitment to place yourself on your yoga mat. The heat component is equivalent to two things: directing your concentration, which is an elegant definition of discipline, and tolerating the discomfort of your own restlessness, which will occur, much like the water experiences in the teapot. Thus the science of yoga will better serve you if you (1) provide yourself with proper structure (yoga class, yoga mat, meditation cushion), (2) commit yourself to not entertaining your distracting and dissipating mental broadcasts, and (3) withstand the friction of this discipline. Remember, one of the definitions of fervency is the fiery transformation that arises from the friction of discipline.

FERVENCY YOGA POSES

Structure + Heat = Transformation

These poses require focus, concentration, patience, and commitment. These are the elements that strengthen the contain-ability of our mind. As such, they are also the source of mental heat. When applied lovingly, we get structure plus heat, resulting in transformation.

SIDE WARRIOR POSE

This is a standing pose that builds stamina, concentration, and willingness.

1. Stand with your feet about three feet apart.
2. Turn your right foot out, parallel to the long edge of your mat, and your left foot in slightly. (This can also be done without a yoga mat, in your sneakers or other street shoes, in the grass, on the pavement, in your office.)
3. Sweep your arms out at shoulder height and stretch them from the center of your chest into your fingertips. Expand through your chest.
4. With an exhale, bend your right knee to 90 degrees. Your shin is best positioned so it is vertical. Your thigh may or may not be parallel to the floor. Your heel ought to feel grounded.

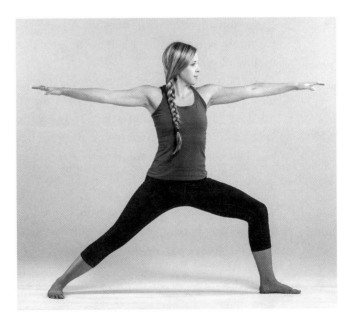

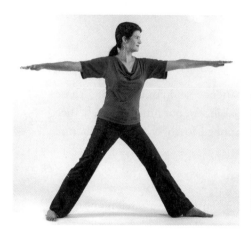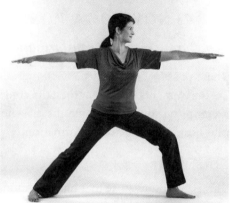

5. Lift your pubic bone up toward your belly button and root your tailbone down toward the floor.

6. Breathe into your belly and commit your mind to experiencing your body. Restrain the urge to think, plan, review, or comment.

7. Concentrate on feeling your feet on the ground, the sensation of stretch in your legs, and the movement of breath in your belly. Restrain the urge to critique yourself. Restrain the urge to dissipate your experience through mental distraction.

8. Keep your attention concentrated on your feet, the stretch sensations, and the movement of the breath. Become an audience to this amazing concert of physiology.

9. If you're trying this pose after recently engaging in disordered eating behaviors or are experiencing a "shame storm," you will need to apply greater fervency to this practice. Deepen your breath and be more forceful with keeping your mind present to you and your body.

10. Stay in the pose for one minute. Then repeat on the other side.

TREE POSE

This is a one-leg balance pose that builds patience, balance, and stillness.

1. Balancing on one leg, lift the other foot and place it high on the inner thigh of your standing leg (or along the inner edge of your leg, perhaps even the inner ankle).

2. Press the foot against the opposite thigh, and your thigh back against your foot.

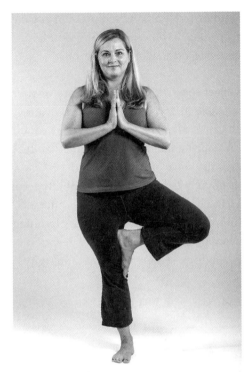
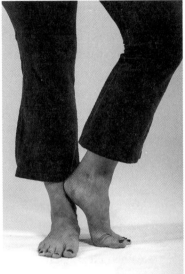

3. Lift your pubic bone and root through your tailbone. Tone your belly.
4. Place your hands at your heart in Anjali mudra.
5. Focus your eyes and explore your balance for one minute.
6. Repeat on the other side.

Discipline as Intuition

Along with approaching the scientific side of discipline, with a foundation of wise humility, we can also engage your desire for a yielding, intuitive reciprocity with your body's journey in recovery. Often, even if we've longed for a more free and fluid approach to "discipline," we've been more fearful of its seeming open-endedness. Women tell me that if they aren't told what to eat, they won't know; that if they don't count calories, they'll lose control; and that if they were to eat intuitively (i.e., listening to what their body craves), they either wouldn't be able to figure that out or they would never stop eating Oreos.

Remember, discipline as intuition relies on wise humility: yoga teaches us that there is an innate intelligence in all things, including your body and your appetite. How, then, do we cultivate a trustworthy intuition?

- By cultivating constant respect for the innate intelligence of your body. If it makes the idea more palatable to you, think of it as cultivating constant respect for the innate intelligence of *nature as represented by* your body.
- By decreasing the noise of your mental broadcasts (the habitual, shame-driven ones) so you can hear the voice of your intuition.
- By increasing the strength of your right hemisphere's ability to push your intuitive voice up to the surface (it has been a bit buried, after all).
- By responding with wise humility, not impulsivity. Your physiology will be your litmus test: am I moving from wise humility and deep respect for nature, or is this my addiction in disguise moving from impulsivity?

FERVENCY: IMPROVISATION + REFLECTION = INTUITION

When I learned to play the trumpet, I was classically trained: I could read and recite music from any of the great composers. I could also successfully play in duets, quartets, or orchestras. I knew the notes and I knew how to use my body as an instrument for music (fingers, mouth, breath, and focus) in conversation with those notes, the conductor, and the other musicians. However, I did not know how to improvise.

Learning to improvise would become an essential life tool for my recovery. To discover, and then be willing to respond to, the voice of my intuition became lifesaving for me. You may recall, another definition of fervency is a fiercely loving, intense commitment to self-awakening. Though I was initially afraid of improvisation, I instinctively knew my recovery, and life at large, would require it. Because I did not know how to improvise with my trumpet, I turned to other means: yoga, art, and poetry. The yoga I'll outline for you in a moment. For art, I purchased blank canvases and watercolor paper and I set about painting as a process without a destination. Sometimes I would look at the blank slate for a long while before a color would choose itself. I had to repeatedly resist the urge to follow thoughts about painting a flower or a house. I waited until I felt the colors choosing themselves. And then I followed whatever curve my hand would take with the brush. Often shapes and color tones would reveal themselves as I went along. At times I would sit quietly again with my canvas in process. I often had to impose a kind of fierce resistance on self-critical thoughts about how poorly I was doing the art or how "stupid" it was going to look. On days when I couldn't find my creativity or my intuition, days when I felt stuck, or even on days when I felt angry or sad and didn't have old coping mechanisms as options anymore, I resisted walking away. I would start with drawing a scribble. It could be a sharp, black, angry line or a lethargic, blue downward slope. The scribble wasn't the end purpose. The scribble was to jog me out of a stuck place and back into my creativity. Once I had a scribble on the page, I would create the next thing off of my scribble. These were often recovery-saving interventions, and I still use "scribble drawing" as a technique with my students today.

FERVENCY YOGA POSES

Improvisation + Reflection = Intuition

For these poses, you're invited to actively improvise. Many of the yoga practices that we use in today's yoga generation are the result of our ancestor yogis feeling their way into discoveries. They were likely improvising, experimenting, and reflecting on the echoes in their body-mind-psyche. To reawaken your intuition, you'll need the same processes.

Reclined Hamstring Stretch

1. Lie on your back with your left leg straight out along the floor and your right leg up with your foot in a yoga strap.
2. This is the basic "canvas" of the pose. Now you get to improvise, experiment, and reflect.
   - You might spread the toes and notice your body's responses.
   - You might experiment with your leg a little straighter or less straight. Feel into what your leg may most want at the moment. Notice any changes in your breathing as a response.
   - You might improvise with how close or far your leg is from your chest.
   - You might also improvise with moving your leg out to the side and observe the responses from your body, breath, and mind.
   - You might experiment with crossing your leg over to the opposite side and observe the responses you get there.

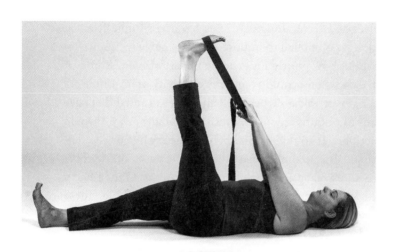

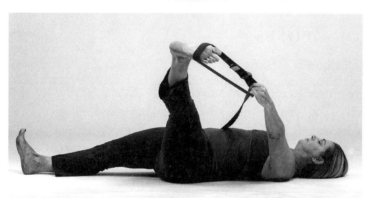

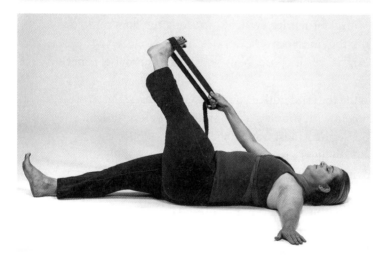

3. In each improvisation (the above are just suggestions), let the instructions be invitations or catalysts. You can explore a few degrees more in any one of them, with the intent to *feel* and reflect on your body's responses.

4. For each improvisation, pause and experience the echo in your body, breath, and mind long enough to really reflect on what's happening. Don't rush to the next suggestion as a linear list of things to do. At each reflection, I invite you to truly wait for the signal from your body about what may be "next" in the artistry of these poses for you.

5. Explore this for two minutes with each leg.

6. Then rest for two minutes.

SEATED DOUBLE-ANGLE POSE

1. Sitting on a blanket or cushion, bring the soles of your feet together.

2. Hold the ankles or toes with your hands and begin with a few deep breaths while sitting up straight.

3. This is the basic "canvas" of the pose. When you feel ready, open yourself to improvising and reflecting on the responses of your body to feel your way into what your body is asking for today.
   - You might explore leaning a bit left or right and listening to your body's responses.
   - You might explore leaning forward into a deeper hip or groin stretch. Play with how far forward you bend, not necessarily determined by your "end

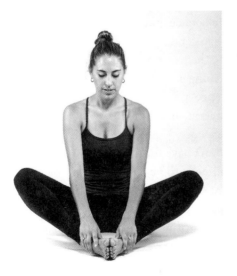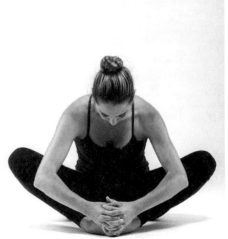

range" in the pose. Play with an attitude of discovery about the process, not the destination.

- You might explore the poses with your feet closer or farther from your hips.

4. In each improvisation, pause for fifteen or twenty seconds to experience the echo in your body, breath, and mind. At each reflection, truly wait for the signal from your body about what may be "next" in the artistry of these poses for you.

5. Release the pose and then sit in reflection for a minute.

Reasonable Guidelines for Respecting Your Body Intelligence and Nourishing Your Life Vitality

If you've felt that you must keep control over your life (left hemisphere thinking) or that you couldn't trust yourself in opening to a more kind and intuitive relationship toward yourself (right hemisphere gift), know that you're not alone and that shame is driving your thinking. To wrestle yourself free from these stances, we come to the fifth aspect of self-nurturing discipline: establishing reasonable guidelines for respecting your body intelligence and nourishing your life vitality. Recovery is an invitation to more and more deeply know yourself at every level, and as you nourish your life vitality, you feed your brain, your heart, your courage, and your capacity.

How do we respect our body intelligence and nourish our vitality? We'll need reasonable guidelines for how to tend to our body-mind-psyche. I've used the word *reasonable* as a prefix to the word *guidelines* because I know that many who struggle with disordered eating patterns also struggle to know what is reasonable or necessary. In the absence of knowing this, people tend to go to extremes and become rigid or domineering in their thinking. Black-and-white thinking doesn't work. Shame doesn't work. With disordered eating patterns, with body-centered self-hatred, we don't have the ability to use a "going cold turkey" approach. Our body will still need to be fed. It will still be the place we reside. It will still need movement of some kind. Therefore, we'll need to look for a "middle path" approach. Being reasonable is going to develop your life skills more effectively than rigid, all-or-nothing thinking anyway. So as much frustration as you may have (and believe me, I had my own!), if you can

~e Reasonable Guidelines

I want to be *cured*. I am sick of identifying with this illness. I am not going back to bingeing all of the time. I will make it out of this hole of suffering. I am trying so hard to get my body back to a healthy equilibrium. It is so difficult to take care of the body that I am afraid of and that I don't particularly like some of the time.

In gratitude for the efforts I am making, I remind myself that

I am currently listening to the dharma talks (discussions by Sarahjoy on the teachings of yoga philosophy) during my two-hour commute to work (ending the isolation).

I am feeling at least some of my feelings and not bingeing them all away for a later day (acknowledge cravings as deeper signals).

I am eating mostly healthy foods, and I am following the recommended times of day to do so (maintain regular mealtimes and maintain blood sugar).

I am keeping hydration and adequate sleep on my radar screen (hydration and deep rest).

I am feeling the air against my skin and remembering that nature includes Me! (air against my skin).

I am trying new things, driving new ways, to help myself increase my change tolerance (getting comfortable feeling uncomfortable [GCFU]).

—Nancy, age 51

consider the skills necessary for recovery as foundational skills for life, too, then you may feel more inspired. The following list sets out some reasonable guidelines for respecting your body intelligence and nourishing your life vitality:

1. Integrate right brain activities into your daily life.
2. Acknowledge hunger and satiation.
3. Identify trigger and nontrigger foods. Acknowledge cravings as deeper signals and needs.
4. Maintain regular mealtimes (don't skip a meal or starve for later).

5. Maintain balanced blood sugar and proper nourishment.

6. Stay hydrated (see Mindful Attention: Increasing Our Ability to Value, p. 87; Unearthing Faith: Creating Personal Buoyancy through Self-Accountability, p. 153; and Dashboarding as a Recovery Skill, p. 197).

7. Prioritize deep rest for both mind and body (see Restoring Your Fuel Tank, p. 183, and Creating White Space, p. 70). Establish healthy sleep routines (see Unearthing Faith: Creating Personal Buoyancy through Self-Accountability, p. 153).

8. Raise your heart rate for twenty minutes each day (see Raised Heart Rate, p. 154; Unearthing Faith: Creating Personal Buoyancy through Self-Accountability, p. 153; and Dashboarding as a Recovery Skill, p. 197).

9. Restore your senses through nature (see Air against Your Skin, p. 154, and Improvisation + Reflection = Intuition, p. 133).

10. Maintain healthy elimination (the obvious, plus laughing, crying, and sweating).

In chapter 5, "Finding Faith, Reviving Courage," you'll be invited to resurrect your faith in your body by focusing on hydration, rest, raised heart rate, and air against your skin (guidelines 1 through 4 above), and in chapter 6, "Resilience and Self-Empathy," you'll be introduced to "dashboarding," which includes guidelines 6 through 10. Here, we'll examine guidelines 1 through 4, which relate specifically to the desire-discipline pendulum, so that we can undertake them as daily practices from a place of self-nurturing (not self-punishing) discipline.

Integrate Right Brain Activities into Your Daily Life

Integrating right-brain-hemisphere activities into your daily life builds your brain's pliability, adds alternative coping mechanisms to your tool kit for managing stress, and creates invaluable reconnecting opportunities between you and you. When we immerse ourselves in creativity, it lights up parts of our brain associated with intuition, the subconscious, childlike wonder, and joy. Some activities my students and I recommend include collaging, gardening, quilting, painting (even finger painting), coloring (coloring books aren't just for children anymore!), jigsaw puzzles, singing, playing a musical instrument, papier-mâché, felting, pastels, writing haiku or playing with poetry, sand painting, playing with clay, or, as mentioned above regarding my own recovery, scribble drawing. Choose something that is portable and accessible for an

> ⁓ Hunger: a sensation of lightness in the stomach, including the qualities or conditions of craving, rumbling, physical restlessness for body-mind fuel, or mental distractedness about food. If hunger goes untended to and passes into starvation or excessive emptiness, you may also experience shaking, agitation, heightened sensitivity, increased distractedness, and food urgency.
>
> Satiation: a sensation of being filled, satisfied, accompanied by feelings of contentment and the condition of noncraving. If you pass satiation to bloating or excessive fullness, you may experience numbness, tightness, physical pain, difficulty breathing into the belly, or feelings of physical denseness.

easily integrated daily activity. For example, if you choose spinning pottery, that requires some equipment. Collaging requires less equipment and not as much skill. This activity should be a simple activity you can enjoy with a nonjudgmental attitude, and a specific time to nourish the right hemisphere of your brain.

Acknowledge Hunger and Satiation

Because this guideline represents one of the most painful aspects of disordered eating experiences, it's worth a careful conversation. When it comes to your body, appearance, weight, shape, cravings, appetite, hunger, and fullness, you've probably struggled with knowing hunger and satiation, emptiness and fullness; you may even feel frightened of either end of the spectrum.

We cannot learn about our appetites—for food, life, or love—under a punitive thinking regime, nor can we learn to acknowledge our hunger or satiation. (Since *emptiness* and *fullness* have become words that elicit powerful feelings far beyond their intended function, I use the words *hunger* and *satiation* instead.)

Befriending our body's expression of hunger is one of the cruxes of recovery (see p. 100). Getting to know true physiological hunger may feel like an archeological dig. In this regard, it's wise to move delicately toward our hunger. To shine the support of befriending onto our hunger means that we are, quite literally, making friends with it. Similarly we'll want to befriend our feelings of satiation. These nuances, along with hunger, have been muddled by disordered eating behaviors. For now, we're going to start with learning about our hunger and satiation from our direct experience of our physical body. We'll do this in a relatively light, less provocative way, focused more on information gathering and not at all on right or wrong.

❧ YOGA INQUIRY

What Number Is Hunger? What Number Is Satiation? (GAP)

Pause now for a moment to tune in to your stomach. Drop down from your thoughts, from your head, through your throat, your chest, and your ribs into the actual physical organ of your stomach. Notice any sensations present there. How empty or full does your stomach feel? Are you experiencing hunger or satiation? Is there any rumbling? If you've recently eaten, are there any stomach noises of digestion, such as little gurgles?

I use a process called the "appetite spectrum" with my students as they are relearning how to connect with their appetites. It ranges from 1 to 10, with 1 being absolutely ravenous and 10 being uncomfortably bloated. Within this spectrum, where would you say your stomach is right now? Reflect long enough to pick up any nuances with your physical appetite yet not so long as to overthink it.

This inquiry becomes more automatic and helpful as an actual intervention if you repeat it regularly. To have accurate information for yourself, I recommend you jot down your observations regarding the appetite spectrum for several days in a row. Jot this down upon waking, before interacting with food or eating breakfast, following breakfast, before and after any snacks, before and after lunch and dinner, and once more before bed. This jotting down is to help you get truthfully in touch with your experience of hunger. After three or four days of recording this, you'll have information you can use going forward. Particularly notice any highs or lows, peaks or valleys.

For early stage recovery, I don't recommend that you let yourself get into states of hunger that are lower than 3 or states of satiation that are higher than 7. You need to re-regulate your appetite, balance your brain chemistry, and develop your ability to work within reasonable guidelines, not all-or-nothing thinking.

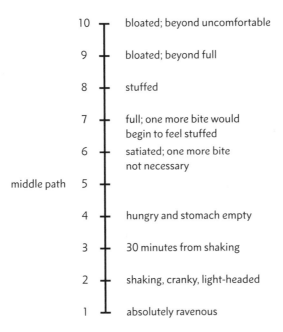

appetite spectrum

10 — bloated; beyond uncomfortable

9 — bloated; beyond full

8 — stuffed

7 — full; one more bite would begin to feel stuffed

6 — satiated; one more bite not necessary

middle path 5 —

4 — hungry and stomach empty

3 — 30 minutes from shaking

2 — shaking, cranky, light-headed

1 — absolutely ravenous

Figure 4.1

Identify Trigger and Nontrigger Foods

Invariably, most of the women with whom I have worked have had specific trigger foods, or categories of food. Frequently, sugar is a big component. Carbohydrates are another. Women rarely report bingeing on broccoli or asparagus, though they might binge on Thai noodles with broccoli, or asparagus fried rice. When I refer to a trigger food I mean foods that stimulate you to keep eating, to emotionally eat all day, to start a binge, to start a cycle of guilt in relationship to eating, to determine that the day has now "been ruined" and ought to just go downhill until tomorrow. The tricky issue is this: is it the food, or our thoughts about the food?

Trigger foods can cause us to feel agitated, even before we engage with or eat them. I can recall, and I've heard from many women, that the approach to a trigger food includes a physiological rush of excitement, anticipation, dread, uncertainty, fear, and animal-like desire. In these times, we are likely to experience the flight from our best selves, a feeling of being hijacked by the trigger food to a place of disembodied, even robotic, frenzy with the trigger food. Homecoming is an essential, lifesaving tool at this juncture (see p. 103). To stay embodied and deeply connected to our best self means staying anchored, at home in our body, and committed to our recovery.

Acknowledge Cravings as Deeper Signals and Needs

To forge a solid recovery, we have to come into relationship with craving. I've talked about disordered eating behavior as a robotic alien invasion. And I recognize that that is truly how it feels. We go robotic. We feel the alien invasion of "that other me" or "the one who can't stay in control." These patterns shrink the circumference of our 360-degree life.

One of the first steps is to acknowledge that a craving is a valid signal: we are responding to a real physiological need, such as for immediate fuel; to a real physiological desire, such as when sugar perpetuates sugar cravings; or to emotional, mental, psychological, olfactory, or visual cues. Coming into relationship with what we crave, how and why we crave, and the nuances of our relationship to craving empowers us.

Sometimes our cravings are driven by a nutritional deficiency, such as when we have cravings for fats, salt, or quick-energy carbohydrates. If you seriously restrict your fat intake, you may be missing the essential, healthy fats. If your electrolytes are out of balance, you may crave salt. And if you're starving yourself of all carbohydrates, you may create a tremendously powerful body-centered directive toward carbohydrates (which whole grains might have satisfied, but when you get to a certain point of hunger and deficiency, French bread or scones look a lot more appetizing than brown rice does). If you have been practicing specific restrictions or if you suspect your cravings are related to nutritional deficiencies, I strongly recommend you seek out a nutritionist with experience in disordered eating patterns.

Some cravings are emotionally driven and may reflect the comfort foods of our childhood. If you acknowledge the drive behind these cravings, you can create a relationship with your valid need for comfort. You can even create a relationship with your inner child's need for comfort and find ways to soothe her that may include food or other calming activities. Acknowledging that cravings can be driven by underlying emotional needs that are valid is very liberating because we come to realize that essentially *all behaviors reflect valid needs.* The trouble is when one behavior obliterates our ability to explore an equally important and valid need. To explore this further, visit my website www.sarahjoyyoga.com for an activity page called "Behaviors, Feelings, Needs, and Strategies."

If you're struggling with cravings driven by olfactory or visual cues, I recommend reading *Mindful Eating* by Jan Chozen Bays. She discusses a variety of ways hunger shows up.

Maintain Regular Mealtimes

If you've been using a strategy of skipping or postponing meals, learning to maintain regular mealtimes may cause you to feel uneasy. Yet, perhaps if you understand the way skipping or postponing contributes to the cycles of painful behavior, you may feel inclined to create more stable mealtimes. For example, it is well researched that dieting that includes calorie restriction becomes a setup for bingeing. Skipping one meal does not set us up for a healthy experience at the next meal.

In the battle to control what you eat and how many calories you consume, your negotiation-based thinking can only become body-disconnected behavior. It is a setup for the disordered eating behavior to win and to become dominated by thoughts about food, calorie counting, dieting, and weighing and measuring. You ultimately become prisoner to this cycle and disconnected from the natural intelligence of the body as a wise and adaptive organism.

Addressing this guideline based on blood sugar, metabolism, and brain function is a skillful way to embark on the efforts to change your meal rhythms. Reducing calories to the point where the body interprets it as a period of famine affects your body's ability to metabolize and absorb the fuel you do feed it. Your body will slow down how it burns calories, and from where it burns them (muscle or fat). You can't run a car with an empty gas tank, even if you're planning to fill it to the brim later that night. Reasonable guidelines for your meal plan can be nutritionally and emotionally safe, especially when created with a naturopath or nutritionist sensitive to disordered eating patterns.

Maintain Balanced Blood Sugar

Similarly, I strongly recommend you work with a nutritionist or naturopath who has direct experience with disordered eating patterns and who can work with you in a profoundly nonshaming way. The scope of this book isn't meant to address the myriad ways in which blood sugar gets out of balance, nor the many useful strategies for consistently bringing your blood sugar back into balance. Yet I can comment through the lens of yoga that all of our systems are interactive means to the goal of health. When we promote health, we experience health, and vice versa. A minor nudge in the direction of health is worth more than it may appear. A minor nudge toward health is also a nudge away from its opposite!

Some factors that may affect your blood sugar include impaired insulin secretion; a stressful or sedentary lifestyle; cellular insulin resistance; being overweight; a family history of type 2 diabetes; a diet high in saturated fat, sugar, and refined carbohydrates and low in fiber; and a diet high in stimulants such as tea, coffee, colas, chocolate, or alcohol.

Some of the symptoms of out-of-balance blood sugar can include needing more than eight hours of sleep, feeling thirsty, needing coffee or tea to get you going, frequent urination in the morning, heavy sweating during the day, fatigue, dizziness, mood swings, cravings for sweet foods, headaches, heart palpitations, and energy dips.

Following through on these guidelines sets the stage for you to experience yourself as worth caring for, teaches you the skills with which to nourish yourself, and increases your self-nurturing discipline skills, giving you the fortitude for the next phase of your journey: finding faith and reviving courage. You're well beyond the trailhead now and, with faith and courage, you'll be able to hike past the familiar switchbacks where you've gotten stuck before.

Part Three

SELF-EMPATHY
(STAGE TWO)

5

FINDING FAITH, REVIVING COURAGE

A S WE DISCUSSED, SWINGING BACK AND FORTH between unhealthy desire and unhealthy discipline, between bingeing and coping, does not lead to recovery. Swinging back and forth becomes disappointing and exhausting. And sadly, it can convince us that we're too undisciplined to get ourselves out of this mess. I know how profoundly frustrating it is to finally convince yourself that "today is the day" when your recovery will begin, when you won't eat those "terrible" things again, only to have it all fall apart in a mystery moment of despair. Yoga sees this despair in terms of buried faith and dissipated courage.

This is the very juice of what this chapter is about: faith and courage, the fundamentals of self-empathy. The ever-swinging pendulums of commitment and breaking of commitment, good days and bad days, indulgence and penance have caused us to lose faith in ourselves, weakened our courage, and narrowed our bandwidth for living a full, 360-degree life.

Shame has had the power to override our original capacities for faith and courage. Through years of exposure to shame (both our original exposures to shame and our repeated self-shaming habits), grooves of doubt, lethargy, fear, and restlessness become embedded into our mind and psyche. This stage of recovery is, in a sense, a very fine archeological dig, where we remove the sedimentary layers caused by shame to unearth the treasures of faith, courage, and capacity. It is also the process of treading new ground, figuratively and literally.

sedimentary layers

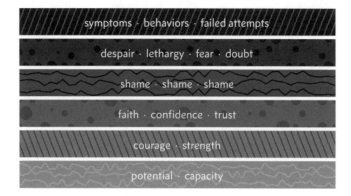

symptoms · behaviors · failed attempts

despair · lethargy · fear · doubt

shame · shame · shame

faith · confidence · trust

courage · strength

potential · capacity

Figure 5.1

What's been buried under layers of sedimentation has an inherent power. It is a power that shame doesn't want us to know about. Shame keeps us buried, frozen, or stuck in the mud. Yet we can call on the power of that which is more deeply buried than the layers of shame as a catalyst for getting unstuck. Long ago we buried our faith and courage, the process of which I'll discuss in a moment. One thing that's critical to understand, however, is that we buried them as a protective measure. Had we been able to express our intrinsic faith or courage, it might have made important people, people responsible for our well-being or safety, uneasy. Had we had the keenness of faith in our body or the boldness of our courage, we may have spoken up, acted out, put up a healthy boundary to harmful behavior, or maintained our healthy appetites, natural body expression, and physical curiosity, as well as our freedom, playfulness, and spark. However, had we done this at the time, it wouldn't have saved our lives. It may have put us in greater danger of harm, isolation, rejection, punishment, pain, or neglect. And, in some cases, we also knew that the risk to try, while it may not have produced outright harm, would have been futile. Rather than bring on the painful disappointment of this, we gave up trying.

Because what we've grooved in the brain has become so magnetically powerful, so deeply worn, and so familiar, we don't realize we're stuck in a switchback of our own making. We're like hikers on a mountain path traversing the same switchback repeatedly. Here in Oregon, we have a lot of mud in our ancient forests. (It rains here!) When we go hiking in the winter, we get a real sense of how slippery, icky, and deep this mud is. You can literally see how many other footprints have come before your own, further deepening the rut in the pathway. Of course, as we're hiking, we can take careful, often playful, steps around these muddy ruts. It's part of the adventure. But when it comes to our minds, we don't tend to see these muddy, rutted switchbacks for what they are. It's confusing because in one direction our switchback looks like conviction, progress, and optimism. In the other direction, it looks like failure, disappointment, and frustration. Again. And again. And again.

This deep grooving is possible only when we've long ago left the mountain trail of faith in our body and courage in our heart. The good news is that the acts of finding our faith and reviving our courage offer us new steps out of the grooves we've been in. Faith and courage will, literally and figuratively, lead us to higher ground.

Faith: a feeling of deep confidence in our journey and our personal commitment to ourselves.

Courage: the strength to take the steps needed on the journey.

Buried faith: currently buried under layers of sedimentation, like the water table available for tapping for a deep well.

Dissipated courage: lost in the frenzy of life, dissipated, like the leaks in a garden hose, in too many unhelpful directions.

How We Lost Faith in Our Body and in Our Recovery

There are two important facets of faith: faith in our body (the faith that our body knows best what it needs when we wisely listen to it), and faith that with the right tools applied, we can recover, even after years of struggling. Both are necessary to healing. We'll look first at how we lost faith in our body, because this loss predates the behaviors we developed that are today's painful cycles. Then we'll look at how we've been losing faith in our ability to recover. In both cases, we'll also talk about what to do and how to regain faith in our bodies and in ourselves.

Tamas: *Yoga's Description of Lost Faith*

From the perspective of yoga, there are energetic manifestations in all of nature. We see it in the way different weather patterns and different creatures express themselves. *Tamas*, one of these energy forms, provides structure and can be stable, grounding, and earthlike.

In fact, tamas in its healthful energy form, is responsible for structure, steadiness, and containment. Yet tamas, when it is out of balance, becomes inert, sluggish, and stuck. We may experience ourselves like thick mud or dense underbrush. Much like the earth's sedimentary layers reveal geological history, our personal history is also layered into our minds and bodies. Yoga refers to our mental sedimentary layers of habit as *samskaras*, underlying patterns that became compulsive, unconscious, and repetitive. These habits are maintained by the momentum of history and familiarity, and create inertia against moving toward the new, the unfamiliar, or the unknown. Addiction is essentially very out-of-balance tamas in which we have become stuck in our behaviors. It is the unalterable nature of addictive behaviors that defines them as tamasic. An important consideration for your thinking about this: we repeatedly turned to these long-overused behaviors as attempts to gain stability.

For recovery, we need healthy tamas, not rigid thinking. We need a fresh foundation, not outdated beliefs. We need deep centeredness, the kind of centering that both comes from and provides us with consistency and integrity. Yet to get there, we must find, underneath our samskaras, our deepest faith in our body's wisdom, like an archeologist digging for treasure.

Losing Faith in Our Body: How Did This Happen?

When you have issues with food, you have the symptoms of a widespread, life-threatening condition: profound disconnection from and loss of faith in your body's intelligence and beauty. This loss of faith began a long time ago. There are many seeds for why and how this disconnection occurs. Perhaps in early life, your body sent messages or signals that were not understood, tended to, or respected by your parents, caregivers, or teachers. These could have been your natural signals for food or water, affection or rest, connection or personal time.

For example, some of my students have described family situations in which mealtimes and food choices were rigidly controlled. A meal was always served at the designated time, always included specific foods, and everyone was always expected to finish everything on his or her plate. Such a rigid relationship to hunger, food, family time, and body rhythms programs a child toward both rigid and rebellious thinking. Rigid thinking comes from internalizing the norms around us. Rebellious thinking arises from the deep creative urge of the individual psyche to resist conformity and manifest itself. In infancy, when conformity is a survival issue, we may conform without actually suppressing this creative urge. In fact, for some of us, as this urge gets compressed into a smaller area of the psyche, the compression makes the creative urge much stronger. This is one reason why we rebel against our own authority from time to time, especially if we set up that authority in a rigid format!

As rigid or rebellious thinking patterns take root in the sea of grown-up voices, needs, and routines, such children would also be required to shut down their faith in their body rhythms and signals about hunger and satiation.

At the other extreme, students have described family situations where the milieu overwhelmingly lacked structure. Mealtimes didn't exist, parents weren't preparing meals, and food was made available at any time, at intermittent but unpredictable intervals, or only by the agency of the child getting food for herself. Routines did not exist; parents were largely unavailable because they may have been too depressed, working too many jobs to keep up at home, or dealing with their own addictions. This kind of chaotic early experience of food and body rhythms does not lay a healthy foundation for an adult relationship to food, hunger, routine, and the body. Yet, by the nature of how our brains develop during the early stages of life, we won't be automatically aware, as adults, that we don't have a healthy foundation. We may not even be able to examine the concept of foundation. We rarely think about the foundation of a house while we are busy reading a book in the upstairs bedroom. In our psyche, what we don't know, or can't examine, hinders us in developing a new and healthy foundation for life.

Another provocation for losing faith in the body's intelligence is when physical boundaries are violated in early life through privacy issues, physical abuse, sexual abuse, or verbal abuse. These events occur at a time when we're relatively powerless due to our age, size, and vulnerability.

Additionally, we may also lose faith in our body's naturalness when watching other people's eating habits, such as when a parent or other family member overeats or undereats. We may suspect something is incongruent, yet from our vantage point as a child, we can't cognitively know. For example, when Mom never eats dinner but always makes it for us, we are getting confusing messages about appetite. "Mom doesn't have an appetite or doesn't need to eat.

Should I?" "Mom is protecting her 'size' or her appearance. Should I do that?" Or, Dad overeats while watching TV news, sports, and such. When we see, and probably feel, a disconnection between physical hunger and "snacking," we internalize this into our body culture as well.

Finding Faith in the Body through Yoga

To overcome out-of-balance tamas, our sedimentary layers of shame and habit, we must create a consistent and strong foundation. We need to leverage the healthy side of tamas that supports our steadiness and grounding. We need to learn how to get still, how to create the consistency that our brains have hungered for, and how to acclimate to the benefits of a healthy foundation. We also need to learn how to tolerate disruptions, to experience turbulence without losing our foundation.

For many of us, we've tried to recover on hope. Hope for thighs to be a certain shape, hope for weight to be a certain number, hope for escaping our shame, hope of not being found out, hope of being loved in spite of our self-loathing, or hope of making it through this day with a little less pain than yesterday. But we aren't going to recover by having hope in intangibles, or hope in the response of others to suit our budding recovery. (If we are so blessed as to have the understanding and support of others, all the better. Yet many people won't have this kind of support. And some may determine this lack of support to be the cause of their relapses.) It is faith in ourselves, faith in our word to ourselves, faith in our willingness to try, and faith in our intelligence, self-worth, and deservedness that will propel our recovery out from under the sedimentary layers of shame, habit, and history.

The practices of yoga clear the mind and give us a glimpse of fresh thinking and faith in life. Because the practices also clear habitual patterns of body stress and disconnection, we'll be waking up not just the muscles and bones, but the underlying archeology of our very selves. Remember how I suggested that shame has been compounded into sedimentary layers, composed of doubt, lethargy, fear, and restlessness? Yoga helps us dig down through these layers to the treasures of our faith and capacity. To dig down, we have to make consistent effort.

To begin the process of finding faith, choose a few clear, body-centered action-steps and commit to them. Faith is rediscovered through making realistic commitments to recovery, rather than black-and-white, desperation-filled, shame-induced commitments. Remember, the fact that you've had the energy to rebel against this kind of discipline is, on the one hand, a sign that your underlying spark is still in there: you know you don't want to succumb to the life-sucking power of shame. On the other hand, this rebellion is also you rebelling against your own recovery. At this juncture, we don't want to set ourselves up for this kind of rebellion. The healthy rebellion of recovery is the rebellion against what has been, against the unhealthy aspects of tamas. What we need is faith in ourselves, the kind that forms as we steadily accumulate moments, hours, days, and weeks of recovery.

YOGA INQUIRY

Unearthing Faith: Creating Personal Buoyancy through Self-Accountability (PB)

Self-accountability will unearth your faith in yourself. And it's practical. These action-steps require no special equipment, are relevant to anyone for healthy, daily life functioning, and will improve your ability to have faith in your body. With tapas (discipline) in the form of self-accountability you build the consistency and structure that benefit your body and your mind for the journey of recovery. Additionally, this healthy structure is in fact the healthy structure of tamas: the structure that stabilizes you on your journey.

REST

- Set a consistent bedtime, in order to satisfy your brain and body's needs for deep and proper rest. I want you to be able to wake up feeling refreshed in the morning!
- Set a consistent wake-up time. (Yoga recommends we wake up with the sunrise.) Even if you have an inconsistent schedule, a consistent wake-up time is going to help you establish healthy routines. You won't need to be on this schedule forever (the dreaded "forever" that causes us to jump off the path of these kinds of decisions!). However, in the early stages of recovery, consistency builds your foundation for recovery. Do what you say you're going to do and you will start to trust yourself again. Deciding nothing would be an easy out but wouldn't give you the chance to build your self-accountability muscles.

HYDRATION

• Commit to drinking the amount of water your body needs to be hydrated. In today's world, this has become an act of radical self-care. (Generally, the amount of water your body needs is, in ounces, the number resulting from your body weight divided by two. If you exercise, you'll need more water.)

RAISED HEART RATE

• Commit to twenty minutes a day of an activity that raises your heart rate. This can be as mild as a walk around the block or as vigorous as you like. This is not to count calories burned but rather to make a commitment to clearing your mind and body through raising your heart rate and getting some deep breathing into your system. In the beginning of recovery, please limit this to twenty doable minutes. For your recovery, I'm also asking you for yoga-based commitments that will require you to create the time to do them. You cannot "squeeze it all in" to your life and have it be effective. Additionally, overexercising also comes with its own health and weight problems. (This is a topic that is beyond the scope of this book.)

AIR AGAINST YOUR SKIN

• Commit to twenty minutes a day of having the air against your skin. You might sit outside in nature, walk slowly in your neighborhood, or take in the night sky from your porch. This is a meditative endeavor. I want you to feel the air against your skin as life's invitation for you to belong. As humans we forget something essential: we are a part of nature, just like the trees and wild animals. To feel the air against your skin is to feel life calling you out of isolation and habit into an experience of belonging and freshness.

If you're already doing all of these things exceptionally well, check to see if your relationship to these activities is based in love and self-accountability or shame and self-control. If it is the latter, I recommend two things: First, set an attitude of tremendous self-care behind each of these commitments. Say it to yourself with everything you do. Remember the power in the exercise Mindful

> ~~~ *Anxiety and Air against My Skin*
>
> I didn't realize what was at the root of my anxious and saddened state until I forced myself out of the house this morning and got some fresh air. After I cleared my head, I realized how much sadness I still have around my relationship with my family. I'm realizing how difficult it is to stay properly inflated when I have so many family members who drain my resources instead of helping me replenish them. I'm doing my best to make choices around food, hydration, rest, e-mail, texting, and my social time to help me stay properly inflated.
>
> *—Jackie, age 36*

Attention: Increasing Our Ability to Value (p. 87). Through this you will raise the volume on the self-respect voice. Second, add one profoundly nurturing thing to your self-accountability tool kit: for instance, take a hot bath or do fifteen minutes of savasana every day.

You'll notice that not one of these is a food-centered suggestion. The only food-centered suggestions that I'll give you in this book appear in the discussion of self-nurturing discipline, which you read in chapter 4. My hunch is that most of us have tried reorganizing our diet as a means to recover, without looking at the balance of ways in which we provide fundamental nurturance to ourselves. Remember the sound panel as a recovery metaphor? This is where we raise the volume knob of self-accountability by committing to practices of rest, hydration, heart rate up, and air against skin, while lowering the volume knob of obsession with what, how, and when we eat.

Losing Faith in Our Ability to Recover: How Did This Happen?

The second aspect of faith that needs to be renewed is faith in our ability to recover. During all the times we've made agreements with ourselves and then broken them, we've been setting ourselves up to lose faith in our ability to recover. Broken commitments, postponement of healing, and shame cause the pain of self-abandonment and rejection. We can't recover while in this state of disconnection. Additionally, this experience of lost faith in ourselves about our ability to recover will produce two significant, but repairable, things: a whirlwind mind searching for strategies, and systemic tension in the mind and body. Loss of faith, conscious or not, activates psychological, mental, and physiological patterns, all of which lead to repetitive cycles of unmanageable food episodes.

Through my recovery twenty-five years ago, and my work with women over the past fifteen years, we've come to describe these confusing and painful cycles like this: *it* feels like it is happening *to us*. The disordered eating feels like a "robotic, alien invasion" where we are no longer our intelligent, deliberate self but rather are swept along by forces we can't see, yet which we feel mightily. These unseen yet powerful forces transport us through the patterns of our behaviors, whether it's a sugar binge, manic chocolate attack, alcohol and cigarettes, or ice cream and popcorn. We have the feeling of being overtaken by a mysterious (yet familiar) force, which makes us move about in haze-like fashion or in a frenzy, repeating steps we could do in our sleep. It can last an hour, three hours, a day, or days and days in a row. The powerful thing to recognize is that it feels like *it* is happening *to us*!

From this perspective, we experience ourselves as helpless and powerless to change the patterns. Life becomes a series of strategies for preventing, managing, and recovering from these robotic episodes. When we've been in the cycles of addiction, we've grown accustomed to living in reaction to our addiction: we seek prevention strategies, we seek recovery strategies, we seek strategies for maintaining secrecy, we seek strategies for keeping those aspects of our addiction that we like and expelling those aspects that we hate. Life literally becomes a series of strategies for preventing, managing, and recovering from our addiction. This has a profound impact on our body, mind, and heart, and creates a kind of frenzy that has us feeling anything but grounded.

Finding Faith in Our Ability to Recover: Using Our Yoga Tools

When we watch a kite sailing in the sky, most of us are drawn to the dance of the kite itself. We watch how it floats, dives, sails, rises, falls, and swoops along. In the process of addiction, we've likely already experienced times where we feel more like a kite in a windstorm than a skillfully soaring kite. In recovery, we will need to know how to skillfully experience floating, diving, rising, falling, and swooping. This is where the life skill of getting in the GAP

✏ *Not Just Being Smarter*

It is critically important to understand that you will not be able to overcome the forces of the robotic alien invader by simply trying to outthink it or yourself. It is not a matter of just being smarter next time. The forces are too powerful. Your behaviors have been too practiced. You will need specific skills to combat the robotic alien invader that, surprisingly, is attempting to come to your aid to alleviate whatever despair you are (or could be) experiencing. As strange as it sounds, this well-trained robotic, alien invader has become so adept that it will even try to "protect" you from yourself as you attempt to move your recovery forward. This happens because recovery, and all the processes associated with recovery, require you to take risks toward a more balanced, competent, fulfilled, and contented life. To your little invader, those risks and their prospects will look terrifying!

becomes critical. To explore this, we're going to use a yoga tool that I call "tracing the kite string." This exercise is one of the basic steps we can take to regain power over the robotic, alien invasion and to profoundly restore our nervous system.

YOGA MINDFULNESS MOMENT

Tracing the Kite String (GAP)

Tracing the kite string, an iteration of Getting in the GAP, is the process of moving our attention off the kite, the wind, the torrents of helplessness, self-hatred, confusion, or despair, and back down the kite string to the ground where we're holding the reins. We visualize this process to train our brain to loosen its grip on the kite itself and to strengthen our tamas, our healthy groundedness.

In the exercise, we move our attention from the kite tossing about in the winds of life down on the kite string, down and down and down (getting grounded), until we feel our hand holding the reins. And then we hold our attention right there. Right there. Right there. Of course the mind will jump back up to the kite, repeatedly, ferociously, unconsciously, habitually. Here is a piece of really good news: your mind has practiced going back to the kite countless times. That's why its habit is so well developed — because you practiced it. Repeatedly. Your mind can practice *not* going back to the kite! You can learn to hold its reins in your hand (paying attention). Tracing the kite string, in yoga, is the skill of experiencing strong sensation in a yoga pose and training your mind to trace the mental kite string of reactivity down and down to the place where you simply make contact with what is occurring in the here and now (as you read, do yoga, or live your life!), inevitably discovering your sense of steady presence.

TEMPLATE FOR TRACING THE KITE STRING (GAP)

- Sensations lead to mental reactivity.
- Lift attention off the windy kite mind and trace the kite string to ground attention down to your fingerprints, heels, toes, yoga mat, sensation alone.
- Keep grounding, grounding, and grounding again into the present moment of this immediate physical touchstone of sensation.
- Sensation rises again. A rush of heat, a change in heart rate or breathing, or a surprising feeling of lightness in the heart leads to mental evaluations: Is it pleasurable? Painful? Safe? Frightening? Right? Wrong? Welcomed? Unwelcomed? Good? Bad?
- Without awareness, the windy kite mind swings back and forth among windstorms of experience, evaluation, desire, and aversion.
- Lift attention off the windy kite mind and trace the kite string to ground your attention.
- Distraction arises: The mind jumps back to the kite. The mind quickly scans for relief — ways to avoid pain, feel pleasure, feel good, get numb, escape, or get control over our experiences.
- This leads to a life overruled by the windstorms.
- Lift attention off the windy kite mind and trace the kite string to ground your attention, again and again, as often as needed to train your tracing-the-kite-string mental muscles.

To trace the flush of yoga sensations back to the ground, to trace the kite string down to our immediate experience, requires concentration and commitment. Yoga calls these *dharana* and *abhyasa:* concentration and willful effort. Once we find ourselves making contact with the tangible here and now of our physical experience, of our hand holding the kite string, a surprising thing will occur: the mind will start to quiet down, thought will slow down, and reactivity will be less capable of pulling us back into the windstorm. With this, we have begun the process of mindful mastery over our reactivity as well as mindful mastery in our response to or within the winds of life. We are becoming present.

YOGA MOMENT

Tracing the Kite String: Restoring the Nervous System (PB)

Healthy tamas, or structure, relies on, and returns great benefit to, a soothed, centered, and refreshed nervous system. It may be hard to know when your nervous system is disrupted, especially if you've come to know anxiety as your normal state. A disrupted nervous system, from the perspective of yoga, may show up as racing thoughts, a windy kite-like mind, irritability, a tendency toward mental confusion, or feelings of restlessness, to identify some common symptoms. If you live with these things now, consider that your nervous system may need some restoration in order for you to think more clearly and kindly, to make wise choices for your recovery, and to direct your energy away from the windy kite and toward the goals of yoga.

This practice will take about eight to ten minutes.

STANDING WIDE LEG FORWARD BEND, WITH HEAD SUPPORT

Forward bends calm the nervous system, as do poses where your head is lower than your heart. This pose is both. Additionally, having your head supported will regulate blood pressure.

Take a wide stance, either on your yoga mat or on a nonslip surface. Bend forward into a hip and hamstring stretch with support for your head. Because most people's heads don't make it to the floor, we support the head with yoga blocks (or a chair, the sofa, or a short stack of stable books). Having your head supported calms the nervous system and quiets the mind. You will also be able to stay longer in the pose, inviting your mind into quieter states.

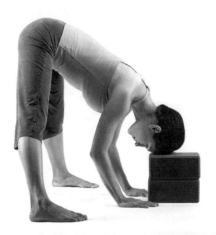
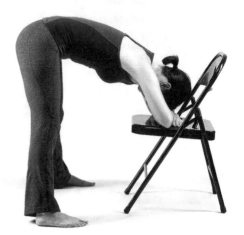

Plan to rest in the pose for one to three minutes. During this time, deliberately trace the kite string down to the physical sensations of where your feet make contact with the ground, how your head makes contact with the support you're using, and how your fingertips experience the floor or the supports you've chosen for them.

Although there will be many other sensations in your body, practice sticking with the bony points that touch the ground. To get in the GAP, we ground our attention to one thing, and then focus attention there repeatedly. You will find yourself arriving in a stronger sense of the present moment. The kite in the sky of the mind may want to generate all kinds of reactions to this pose or to life outside of the pose. Here it becomes critical that you stay more interested in tethering your mind to the present moment, like the hand that holds the kite string, rather than the winds of thought.

- Notice the way your feet make contact with the ground.
- Ground your kite-like mind to just the experience of your toes and heels. If necessary, visualize yourself tracing an invisible kite string from your windy thoughts down into your grounded feet.
- With focused attention, become present to how each toe experiences these moments, including the texture of the yoga mat or floor and the pressure of toes against the ground.
- Notice the weight of your head on the blocks (or alternate support).
- Ground your thinking mind to these specific sensations and become

present to the feeling of your forehead, cheeks, eyes, and jaw all melting away from activity.

- Notice the way your fingertips make contact with the ground.
- Ground your attention to this one tangible thing for this moment of mindful attention.
- Now shift your attention to your breath and place your hands back up on your hips. Inhale and rise up to standing.
- When you come up, promptly put your thinking mind into the bones of your feet, into that which makes contact with the ground. Trace the kite string of any windy thoughts right down through your body and into the floor. Become present to this moment through your experience of heels and toes.

SEATED WIDE LEG FORWARD BEND, WITH HEAD SUPPORT

This pose also quiets the nervous system and supports your body in releasing built-up tension in your hips, spine, or breathing.

If your hips are flexible enough to practice this on the floor, take a seat with your legs stretched out wide. Center a couple of yoga blocks or a stack of pillows (or position yourself with a chair in front of you), and bend forward until your forehead and your arms are supported.

If you're not flexible enough for the floor, or if you simply prefer an accessible setup with common household items, use two chairs. Sit in one chair, facing the other. Step your feet and knees apart so that your knees are wider

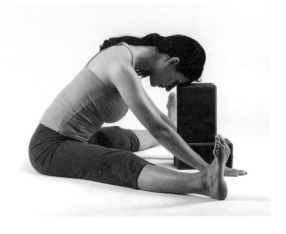

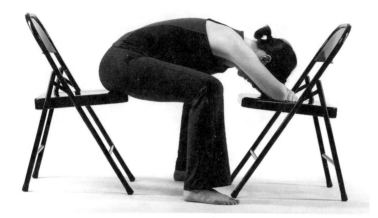

than the seat of the chair in front of you. Bend forward and rest your forearms and forehead on the seat of the chair in front of you. If the chair is too low to comfortably reach, you may use a desktop or table.

Plan to rest in this pose for one to three minutes.

- Notice the way your heels make contact with the ground.
- Ground your kite-like mind to just the experience of your heels.
- Repeat the instructions for tracing the kite string from the first pose.
- When you come up, promptly put your thinking mind into your hip bones, into that which makes contact with the ground or the chair. Trace the kite string of any windy thoughts right down through your body and into the floor or chair. Become present to this moment through your experience of your hip bones.

SEATED *JANU SIRSASANA*, WITH HEAD SUPPORT

Janu sirsasana is a quieting pose that can be done on the floor or with two chairs. On the floor, sit with your left leg stretched out straight and your right leg folded in so that your right foot rests on the floor against your inner thigh. Once more you'll be folding forward, aiming to rest your head on a support. Either set up a stack of blocks or bring a chair close enough to rest your forehead on.

With two chairs, sit in the first chair facing the second. Step your left leg up onto the chair. Keep your right foot flat on the floor, and step your leg out to the side of the chair.

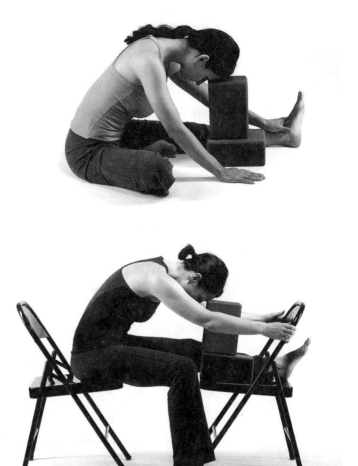

Fold forward to rest your head on a support (like a pillow). If your hamstrings are too stiff for this, put a yoga strap around your left foot and hold it with both hands. Bend forward as far as your body allows you to, and determine how high a support you would need for your head. If you need quite a bit of height, turn around the chair that your left leg is resting on. The back of the chair may be the right height for your head and forearms now.

Plan to stay for one to two minutes on each side.

• Notice the way your feet experience this position differently. Mentally make contact with the ground by focusing on your feet.

- Ground your kite-like mind to just this experience.
- Repeat the instructions for tracing the kite string from the first pose.
- When you come up, promptly put your thinking mind into your hip bones, into that which makes contact with the ground (or the chair). Become present to this moment through your experience of your hip bones.

This sequence of three poses practiced regularly will quiet your nervous system. (You may still benefit from an in-person consultation with a yoga teacher to assess the way you are setting up the poses.)

REVIVING COURAGE

Once you've unearthed your faith, committed to self-accountability, and practiced restoring your nervous system, you've pulled away from the muddy shores of the riverbank into the currents of possibility. It's quite likely that you've pulled away from your tamasic shores before, only to be swept back. Courage is what keeps you on track now. Not an adrenaline-driven courage, which would primarily activate your fight-flight-freeze-submit reactions, but rather a yoga-directed courage. The difference is in your mind-set.

Fear and excitement very closely resemble each other in the human ecosystem. That is why some things that are terrifying are also fun or exciting, such as roller coasters or riding a bicycle very fast downhill. As we revive our courage, we're going to feel both fear and excitement. The challenge is to move ahead in spite of fear and with healthy excitement. The two may coexist. We only need excitement to be 51 percent of the equation for this to be effective.

One of the things common to all recovery is the fear of excitement. Specifically, the what-if fear: what if, as we outgrow old patterns and become excited for new horizons, we get overwhelmed or lose the progress we've gained and slide back farther into despairing territory? An effective way for working with this aspect of recovery is to think of titrating or acclimating along the way. When fear and excitement coexist *and* we still choose to take action, we're reviving our courage. (In fact, if there weren't some amount of fear involved, we wouldn't really need courage.) When fear begins to overwhelm excitement, we wisely step back slightly to gain stability (tamas) and practice tracing the kite string to reinforce our faith in ourselves and to restore our nervous system. Going back is not the same as going backward. It's wise self-care.

It brings new skills and awareness to present-moment recovery challenges. Maintaining faith in your ability to monitor when you need increased self-care, restoration, or mental fortitude will bring tremendous strength to your healthy recovery foundation.

Losing Courage: How Did This Happen?

If you find yourself having trouble making behavior change, setting clear boundaries with others, or consistently sticking with your priorities, or are feeling fear in facing the unknown, first of all, you're quite normal! And second, you've lost your root courage. Again, as with losing faith in our body's intelligence and naturalness, there are many implications as to how we've lost our courage. Perhaps, for example, you had your exuberance "made bad" by people who were uncomfortable with it. Or perhaps your "boldness" got you into unexpected trouble. Alternatively, if your early environments were chaotic, you may have learned to survive by getting smaller; in the face of that chaos and unpredictability, you may have felt powerless, helpless, or both. You might have lost your courage if you experienced shame when speaking up or if taking a stance meant getting clobbered. Perhaps it wasn't directly your experience, but you saw this happen with someone else. Keep in mind that sometimes a person is bold on the outside but not courageous on the inside. You may experience yourself using bold behavior in specific areas, but may not have other options available. Courage is the ability to do something other than what we've been doing. It helps us forge new ground. It is not the same as rebelling in anger or outrage, yet we might experience each of these things as we revive our courage. We may find ourselves rebelling against old ways of being, or being angry at the forces that we've allowed to suppress us for so long (including our own shame and our behaviors). We may be outraged that the loss of faith and courage is so widespread among humans that its epidemic nature makes it look like normal.

Here's a bit of good news: the faith and courage needed for recovery are also catalyzed by the process of recovery. This reciprocity is something you can leverage! Courage is taking the right action in the presence of fear.

Rajas: *Yoga's Prescription for Reviving Courage*

Rajas is the force in nature that supplies motivation, energy, direction, and focus. Because it can become scattered, frenzied, and move more horizontally than vertically, we'll need to know whether we're becoming adrenaline-driven or yoga-directed. To understand the difference between the horizontal and the vertical patterns of rajas, think of energetically pacing back and forth on a mountain switchback. Much energy may be used with little meaningful direction or gain in altitude. That's horizontal in nature. Actually achieving elevation gain, which happens when we move up and out of those switchbacks, is vertically oriented. To move up the mountain, we need healthy rajas. Yoga invites us to grow, to evolve out of stuck patterns. To do so, we need focused energy.

Out-of-balance rajas might manifest as overscheduling, overcommitting, overindulging, and excessive thinking, ruminating, or endless doing. It is frenzied in nature. The risk of out-of-balance rajas is chronic dissipation of our focus, vitality, and purpose. Burnout. Irritation, frustration, and the sense of being overwhelmed. In this state, we have very little ability to think clearly about alternative options for problem-solving, scheduling, or responding to life. When these patterns become chronic, they become so routinized that conscious thought is not required to keep them in play. Subconscious thought patterns drive our behaviors. At this point, even if it looks like high-paced, frenetic busyness, the pattern itself is described as tamasic. A rajasic habit, when repeated enough, becomes a tamasic problem.

The healthy side of *rajas* is its ability to motivate us to move to higher ground, to move with courage and conviction in spite of fear. This involves a measure of coming into relationship with the unknown. And that, for the human mind, requires our courage in the face of fear and excitement.

◦ YOGA INQUIRY

Moving from Love, not Shame: Fear and Excitement (MLNS)

One of your essential life skills is to move from love, not shame. Shame is adrenaline-driven, and can create adrenal response when it's not necessary or helpful. To know whether we are moving from an adrenaline-driven or a yoga-directed response, we look to the body to give us signals. Fight-flight-freeze-submit patterns come with changes in heart rate, breathing, thirst, pupil dilation, and body temperature. In this inquiry, I'll provide you with two breathing practices: one that shifts you into a yoga-directed, open mind-set

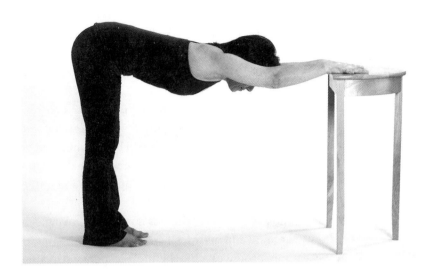

and another, in contrast, that stimulates an adrenal response. Then I'll ask you to repeat the breathing practice that brings you back to your yoga-directed, open mind-set.

INFLATING COURAGE: HANDS ON TABLETOP BREATHING

Similar to the inflating breath practice you learned on page 108, this one has your arms overhead. Yet in this practice you'll be inwardly directed. So this practice inflates your courage while maintaining your connection to your faith in yourself.

Step up to a countertop, desk, shelf, or the back edge of the couch.

Place your hands face down and about shoulder width apart on whatever support you are using.

Step your feet back until your arms and your spine are stretched out straight horizontally from the support. Have a good amount of weight in your feet and heels specifically.

Now, inhale through your nose, slowly and deeply, into your belly.

Exhale, also through your nose, patiently. Imagine a dimmer switch being turned down as you exhale.

With your inhale, breathe broadly into the back hemisphere of your body, where your adrenal glands sit.

With your exhale, turn down the dimmer switch.

Repeat this for six breath cycles.

Step forward toward the support and stand up. Notice how your mind and body feel.

IGNITING ADRENALINE

Similar to the befriending breathing practice in chapter 4 (p. 101), loosely hold your hands behind your back and slightly tip your head forward. Now, deliberately concentrate on taking four to six deep breaths initiated with your chest muscles. Pick up your sternum and collarbones to inhale. Push them down to exhale. Use your upper chest to pump the breath in and out. (This may feel very awkward.)

Then stop. (Stop sooner if it becomes anxiety provoking, which it might.) Notice how your mind and body feel.

Chest breathing produces a biochemical response that stimulates adrenaline.

Diaphragmatic breathing produces the biochemical response of your parasympathetic system, wherein you can experience yoga, openness, and presence.

INFLATING COURAGE, AGAIN

Repeat the first practice, inflating courage, for six breath cycles, as before.

Step back toward the countertop and stand up. Notice how your mind and body feel.

Observe the distinct difference between the outcomes of the two exercises. Because fear and excitement have very similar biochemical expressions, along the path of recovery, it will be very empowering for you to be able to identify if you are in fear or excitement.

Reviving Courage: How Does Yoga Teach This?

We'll need healthy doses of courage to step into the unknown, to step out of our patterns. While restoring faith includes an element of soothing your nervous system through deep quiet, paradoxically, to revive courage, we must take action. We must step out of the pathway of the mountain switchback that we've grooved so well. Having worked with so many women moving toward recovery, I know the trepidation that can arise for people when they are shifting to new and higher ground.

To "revive" something implies a kind of reinvigorating. Let's think in terms of depression versus vitality. Depression is the accumulation of sedimentary layers of disappointment in our ability to act, to generate force, agency, or direction, and to follow through past the initial surge of excitement. Depression is also the proper symptom, from your mind and body, when you chronically experience insight that doesn't turn into action. Because all symptoms reflect the underlying conditions of the body, mind, and heart, the symptoms of lost courage are, in fact, the ones you should be having, given your circumstances, history, and conditioning. For the human psyche, when insight doesn't turn into action, it leaves a sedimentary layer of disappointment and loss of faith in ourselves. When we are able to rouse and direct our energy toward action, we experience a rise in our vitality. Although this process can go unnoticed by our conscious mind, each layer of insight without action leaves a residue, and each moment where insight turns into action builds a bridge out of that residue. It takes tremendous courage to translate insight into action. That's why so many people don't do it!

When you stay attentive to the process of insight, you will start to become more aware of the inner negotiations that you move through in deciding whether this insight will turn into action or not. (Please note that insight is different from impulsivity.) Here are a few examples of common insights women have when stepping onto the path of recovery:

- I can't keep doing this anymore. It is literally killing me.
- I need help.
- What I am doing is not normal behavior. I am at war with my body. I want this to end.
- The way I have been trying to get out of this isn't going to work. It's actually part of the problem. I need to do something new.

These aren't simple insights to turn into action. These are the kinds of insights that require significant energy to move toward action. And that is where we can get paralyzed. When we get paralyzed, we won't feel we have the tools or knowledge to go about the changes that these insights suggest, such as altering the paradigm through which we've been managing our feelings.

✣ YOGA INQUIRY

Getting Comfortable Feeling Uncomfortable (GCFU):
Two Toeholds in the Right Direction

If we break down a big insight into smaller action-steps, we're going to find it easier to make progress and develop some confidence in ourselves. One of the phrases we use in my recovery groups is "two toeholds in the right direction." This is, essentially, four toeholds, if you count the two you didn't take in the "wrong" direction. Two toeholds on the path to recovery is often all you can manage. Yet to manage to sustain it is a courageous thing. You'll have to use your getting-comfortable-feeling-uncomfortable skills for this one, because it is often more uncomfortable to "just stand still" where you are, with those two courageous toeholds, than it is to backslide or try to launch yourself out of the discomfort to who knows where.

When I talk about how this might look with my recovery groups, I use the image of a person standing in a windstorm. When the wind is coming at them, the effort it takes not to slide backward is a real force in the right direction, yet they might appear not to be moving. Similarly, your two toeholds in the right direction may not look like much at times, but incremental steps make up the journey. Even when you appear to be standing still, you're generating the strength to move forward.

Let's go back to insights I mentioned before and look at how your inner language toward those insights might shift to give you some traction away from old ruts and mental switchbacks.

One of the insights was *I can't keep doing this anymore. It is literally killing me.*

That insight implies stopping "everything," which would terrify your system. It would also paralyze you because you wouldn't know where to start. When you feel overwhelmed or confused, these are acute times for getting triggered. Women often find themselves eating because they feel overwhelmed or confused and "aren't sure what else to do."

TWO TOEHOLDS LANGUAGE

Just for this hour (or moment), I will not [binge, purge, starve myself, research another diet].

Just for this moment, I am making this choice in the direction of my recovery.

Just for this hour (or moment), I will not [shame, hate, punish myself].

Just for right now, I turn my toes away from shame and toward recovery.

Just for this hour, I will not weigh myself (or evaluate myself in the mirror).

For this moment, I am exploring two toeholds toward self-acceptance.

Just for this hour, I will courageously withstand discomfort a little longer than I did yesterday.

This is four toeholds away from old behavior.

Just for this moment, I will feel what I am feeling, without making it wrong.

I am four toeholds farther from shame.

Just for this day, I will practice two of the tools I'm learning in this book.

Another insight: *What I am doing is not normal behavior. I am at war with my body. I want this to end.* This insight might have historically kerned you toward black-and-white thinking or rigid plan-making.

TWO TOEHOLDS LANGUAGE

Just for this moment, I realize war won't work.

Just for this moment, I recognize I have been in pain.

Just for this moment, I forgive myself.

For this moment, I am two toeholds closer to recovery based in self-nurturance.

Just for this hour, I am willing to resist all-or-nothing thinking.

I am four toeholds farther from shame.

Just for this day, I commit to two self-nurturing discipline action-steps.

Rajas, as discussed earlier in this chapter, is what fuels our focus, determination, and drive. Even if all we can do is stand still in a windstorm, rajas is still our ally in turning insight into action. It is rajas that helps us resist the fear that prevents us from responding clearly to our insights. Rajas is strength, even boldness, wielded in the right direction. In recovery, this is the direction away from old behavior and toward the new horizons represented by turning the corner on the mountain switchback to rise vertically out of that deeply grooved rut. Rajas is the courage to bravely entertain the questions of your life hunger and move toward your 360-degree life!

❧ YOGA MOMENT

Increasing Personal Buoyancy: Embodying Your Courage (PB)

UPWARD HANDS, CHAIR POSE, AND FORWARD BEND SEQUENCE

Stand with your feet hip distance apart and parallel.

Bring your palms together at your heart. Center your attention in your belly (even if you hate your belly).

Take a deep breath in through your nose. Exhale completely, also through your nose.

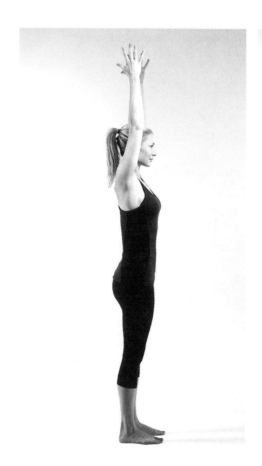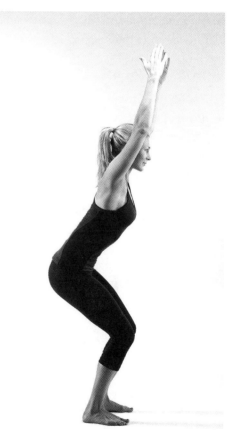

Now inhale deeply again and sweep your arms up overhead. Reach deliberately, strongly, and courageously. Imagine yourself pushing up against the sedimentary residues of insights that didn't turn into action.

Reach beyond the tips of your fingers and feel your heart, mind, and energy rise.

With an exhale, sit down into chair pose: bend your knees, drop your weight back into your heels, root your tailbone, and, as you keep your arms rising enthusiastically, drop your attention in to the strength in your center. This is the strength of your conviction and determination. It is also muscle strength and the strength of your breath, but primarily it is your rajas strength.

Breathe deeply five times.

Then exhale and bend forward to touch the floor (if your hamstrings are tight, keep your knees bent).

This forward bend is a chance to release any fear or doubt about your ability to rise. Inhale and exhale deeply, even sighing on the exhale. In fact, I recommend sighing audibly. It can help release the tension in your throat, belly, and mind.

Then gather your energy into your center again and, with an exhale, bend your knees back into chair pose.

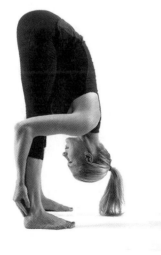 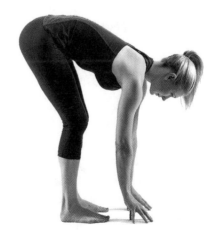

Inhale, and lift your chest, heart, head, and arms into chair pose.

Reach very strongly from your center upward, even while you root down from your tailbone to your feet. Plant yourself firmly in your conviction while at the same time reaching courageously toward your goal.

Take five strong breath cycles here.

Then inhale and rise back up into upward hands pose.

Exhale and bring your palms together at your heart.

Acknowledge the efforts you've made.

Feel the physiological echo of those efforts.

Repeat twice more, deliberately acknowledging the commitment it takes to repeat the exercise. (It takes more effort to repeat this than it does to sit down again.)

Then either stand or sit quietly and witness the vitality expressing itself through your body. You might feel a tingle in your hands, warmth in your legs, or a sense of overall aliveness in your body. Your heart rate and body temperature may be up, yet you can quietly observe your body's intelligence now settling that down to homeostasis. Trust this vital energy to restore your body and clear your mind. One of the blessings of courage is the openness of heart that comes with it.

This practice can be done to revive your courage and commitment at any time. It is energizing and grounding. It requires you to actively participate, but it can be done even when you feel lethargic.

❧ YOGA INQUIRY

Increasing Personal Buoyancy: Embodying Courage in Everyday Life (PB)

There are several other gestures or commitments you can use to embody the rajas of your courage and commitment. These are the gestures of daily life. Here are some examples:

- getting out of bed when you don't feel like it
- taking a shower when you don't feel like it
- stepping out the front door to walk around the block, especially when you don't feel like it

- making a phone call to reach out of your isolation or despair
- turning off the TV or computer, and reducing the impact of these on your mind and body
- doing jumping jacks or jumping rope to overcome the swirling of fear, anxiety, and depression that arises as you contemplate change
- sitting down to eat your meal
- saying no to _____ (fill in the blank)
- keeping your commitment to twenty minutes of raised-heart-rate activity each day
- lifting your chest and heart when mental shame habits start up

Think about what might be on your personal list of things you can do to embody courage.

DISCOVERING LIGHT

The two energy forms called *tamas* and *rajas* are part of yoga's teachings about the *gunas* (meaning "strand"). In these teachings there is a third energy pattern called *sattva*. In recovery, sattva is what happens as a result of finding faith and reviving courage. Through the effort to create an unshakable foundation and the determination to rise in spite of fear, toward the lucid, open, expansive, luminous expression of the undiminished human heart, we discover light. Sattva is the energy form of auspiciousness, lucidity, and grace. We see and feel it in the dusk and the dawn, in the light dappling through the trees, and in the quiet awe of mountain streams. In human nature it is our capacity to live with wise humility, awe, and tenderness, and to be at ease in our innate belonging and wholeness. Sattva is the lucid heart capable of forgiveness and reflective of our innate joy and freedom. You'll be offered meditations for awe, tenderness, belonging, and wholeness in chapter 7, and the teachings on forgiveness and freedom in chapter 8.

6

RESILIENCE *and* SELF-EMPATHY

THE NOUN *RESILIENCE* IS DEFINED BY WIKI-pedia as "the ability of a material to absorb energy when it is deformed elastically, and release that energy upon unloading." The American Heritage Dictionary of the English Language defines *resilience* as "the ability to recover from illness, depression, adversity, or the like; buoyancy" and also "the property of a material that enables it to resume its original form, position, etc., after being bent, compressed, or stretched; elasticity."

For our purposes here, I would like to define *resilience* as our bounce-back-ability; our recover-ability; our personal buoyancy; a blend of our strength and flexibility in mind and body. We could also say that *resilience* is the result of surviving disregulation, discomfort, or disruption without self-medicating; it is the result of not self-abandoning, the result of having faith in ourselves and in life.

We were meant to live with some measure of resilience in life. It is an essential part of how the human species adapts and evolves. To support your recovery, your resilience needs to be restored. The journey ahead will require you to have enough resilience to courageously explore new terrain, withstand the discomfort of change, develop more mental stamina, and respond to periods of doubt with confidence and conviction.

It is very hard to do this well if you don't have the internal resources to meet the demands of life. There are important mental and emotional skills that we need, some that we missed developing along the way when we learned to substitute disordered eating patterns for skills. Our ability to consider, learn, and then integrate new skills will rely on our overall physical well-being. Simultaneously, *our ability to deeply restore our physical health and well-being relies on our ability to address our thinking habits.* Our body-mind-psyche has only so much reserve, so much fuel in the vitality tank at any given moment. It apportions attention to the most pressing demands. For example, when we're exhausted, suffering from a terrible headache, or fighting off the flu, we're much less capable of remembering and utilizing a new life skill. Resources are being directed toward the repair of the physical body. This is why a yoga-based recovery program sees addressing your physical body, which is intimately linked with your mind, as fundamental to recovery itself. Fortunately, addressing your mental habits, including the tone of the inner voice with which you speak to yourself, has a profound reciprocity with your physical well-being. As we move into this discussion, on the foundation of kind self-study, we cultivate self-empathy. It is necessary for us to explore our thinking habits with a heart of tenderness, not an attitude of condemnation.

The biggest drain on our vitality fuel tank is our thinking. Our brain requires the most resources; our thinking causes the most disruption; and then our physical symptoms reflect the drain that our thinking habits cause to our vitality. These drains can be such things as mental anxiety that leads to insomnia, mental habits that lead to food indulgences (or lead to couch potato habits that cause poor digestion), mental tension that becomes chronic muscle aches and pains, or the inner voice tone of shame (about any one of these patterns) that leaves you feeling demoralized. Most of us have been taught to address our physical symptoms only at the level of the physical body (and we may think that if we solve these symptoms, shame will leave us alone). Sadly, we can keep ourselves very busy just trying to keep up with symptom management! More sadly, this symptom-management strategy distracts us from the underlying discoveries at the root of our symptoms. Fortunately, the practice of yoga gives us the direct experience of just how intimately linked our body and mind are. And as yoga does relieve many physical symptoms, we will see this body-mind connection very personally.

The road to recovery involves skills that you can turn to repeatedly in navigating the new terrain of your life and the times when you're feeling less than your best. In the early stages of recovery, restoring your physical vitality will help you have a brain more capable of taking the risks to learn new skills. Restoring your physical vitality with self-nurturing discipline is also

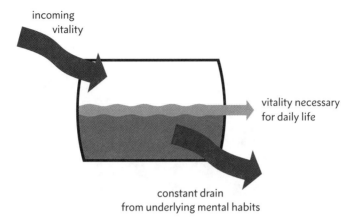

vitality fuel tank

incoming vitality

vitality necessary for daily life

constant drain from underlying mental habits

Figure 6.1

empowering and builds your faith in yourself as a person able to be successful with this. By taking the steps to care for your vitality, you are demonstrating your ability to navigate life wisely, to choose self-respect and self-empathy over shame, and to return to clarity even in the midst of physiological distress. In short, you are building your resilience.

LEAKS IN THE FUEL TANK

When the physical body is in balance, it ingests food, digests food, absorbs what is useful, and eliminates what is not useful. Through this process the body feeds the brain clear fuel—proper nutrients, minerals, amino acids, and fatty acids. (Your brain will work better! Your mind will function more clearly.) Common binge foods include refined sugars, processed carbohydrates, saturated fats, and excessive amounts of each. These are foods that our body, and our brain, has to work harder to "overcome" for clear thinking to take place. In other words, the less a food resembles its whole food components, the more chemicals in the food, and the more nutritionally deficient a food is, the more it drains, rather than gives to, your vitality. Vitality is not the same as a sugar high. The more energy it takes to digest and metabolize binge foods, the more likely you are to be drawing fuel from your reserves. This puts your body into its catabolic, or wear-and-tear, response—and it costs you more than you realize. Simply put, it vastly diminishes the scope of your 360-degree life.

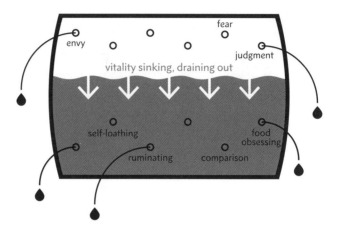

leaks in the
vitality fuel tank

fear

envy

judgment

vitality sinking, draining out

self-loathing

food obsessing

ruminating

comparison

Figure 6.2

To prevent chronic drains on our physical energy and mental clarity, we must understand this: life under the spell of disordered eating patterns, shame-based inner dialogue, or body-centered self-loathing causes countless pinpricks in the fuel tank of thinking, confidence, vitality, and hope; and this causes us to lose focus on adapting, flourishing, and evolving in life. Yo-yo dieting, severe calorie restriction, emotional eating, and compulsive exercise, for example, may have been attempts to regain some control over life, but these strategies don't encourage us to examine our thinking or develop new, healthy life skills. Nor are they just us misbehaving or not having enough willpower. They all arise from mental patterns that we internalized long ago, and that have become automatic thinking habits, that became behaviors and food choices that have dis-regulated our body's natural intelligence. Simply said, the most critical of the countless pinpricks in our vitality come from our thinking. These become much larger than a pinprick, and much more draining, when this thinking comes with the voice tone of shame.

Recovery will require us to think differently. Even though you may experience your thinking as chaotic, unruly, or confused, addiction thinking is actually rigid. Yoga defines rigidity in this regard as unchallenged patterns repeating themselves without interruption, causing a greater likelihood of endless repetition. I like to say it as "thoughts thunk a thousand billion times

∼꧒ *Restoring Vitality through Yoga*

Yoga practice reduces the wear and tear on the body. When you reduce the wear and tear, the body's vitality and capacity are restored. This increases your ability to feel confidence and clarity. As such you will make better decisions with increased courage. This allows you to restore faith in yourself and to build your resilience. You will also develop a stronger and stronger ability to maintain sobriety, with a more and more clear mind. You will naturally become less inclined to cause wear and tear on your body. This will further increase your confidence, clarity, and faith.

without a challenge to newness." Some of the more common thoughts thunk a thousand billion times, related to disordered eating patterns and body-centered self-loathing, include:

"I'm fat!"
"I hate my thighs."
"Tomorrow will be different."
"I deserve this chocolate."
"I'm hopeless."
"Why am I doing this?!"
"I'll start my diet . . ."
"Once I get to . . . then I will be allowed to . . ."
"Forget it. This is too hard."
"I've been good/bad today."
"I need to be thin."
"I'll just do this . . . once more."
"I'll work this off later at the gym."
"I earned this."
"I might as well give in."
"There must be something really wrong with me."
"I can't go to . . . looking like this!"
"This will never work. I give up."
"I am good / bad."

To rebuild our resilience against these kinds of automatic thoughts, we must learn to think differently *and* we must establish some physical sobriety with food. Our moods, thoughts, and feelings are fed by the foods we eat as much as our hips are. For optimal functioning, our brain chemistry relies on specific nutrients in balanced proportions. When we dis-regulate our brain, through poor food choices, bingeing, restricting, overexercising, or under-exercising, even through compulsive thinking about these things, we can't function optimally; we can only function suboptimally. For example, we may be outstanding in our job duties, but at a high cost to the rest of our life. We may even feel we have a terrific life, but our disordered eating patterns won't let us enjoy it.

Just in case you've forgotten how much reciprocity there is among your thoughts, perceptions, reactions, and moods, consider this:

> When you walk by a storefront window and like (or don't like) what you see, your mind, inner voice tone, and body respond . . .
> When you step on the scale and like (or don't like) what the number says, your mind, inner voice tone, and body respond . . .
> When you have a positive interaction with a friend, your mind, inner voice tone, and body respond . . .
> When you practice yoga, your mind, inner voice tone, and body respond . . .
> When you experience empathy, connection, and attunement, the feeling that another person really "gets" you, your mind, inner voice tone, and body respond . . .

Similarly, the thinking patterns that feed your addiction affect your mind and your body. And, as powerfully, a change in thinking patterns can greatly leverage your sobriety and establish a foundation for your recovery.

Every time we commit to rebuilding our resilience by challenging our thinking habits, even if we aren't immediately successful, we're patching up a leak in the fuel tank. Every time we shift our voice tone from shame to self-empathy, we shore up critical leaks in the fuel tank. Likewise, each time we eat foods that nourish rather than deplete or challenge our vitality, we shore up another leak. This is not a quick fix, but done deliberately and consistently, it's guaranteed to change your life. As I said previously, you've already run the experiment you're living. *You know the results of your current thinking — and of your food and diet and exercise choices — on your mind and body, and the impact they have on your life.*

YOGA MOMENT

Restoring Your Fuel Tank (PB)

Yoga's library of poses to use as medicine, for the body, mind, or heart, includes "restorative poses." These are poses done with yoga props to support the body so that we can remain in the yoga pose for a longer duration of time, quiet the nervous system, open the lungs and heart, and allow our digestive, immune, and endocrine functions to come back into balance. These are essential systems to our vitality, but the fight-flight-freeze-submit reaction in the human organism suppresses their function in order to direct resources to managing the emergency at hand, whether it is real or perceived.

Below are two restorative poses for shoring up your fuel tank. The first pose has the legs higher than the head, which sends fresh blood, oxygen, and nutrients to your brain. The second pose opens the belly and the pelvis, reducing stagnation in digestion, elimination, and menstruation. It is also helpful during pregnancy because it lets the pelvis, belly, and uterus rest, while also gently opening the hips.

Please set up carefully, as you will be doing the poses for ten to fifteen minutes.

LEGS-UP-THE-WALL POSE

Position yourself on your side near enough to a blank wall and close enough to the baseboard to scoot in and roll onto your back with your legs resting up against the wall.

Suggestions:

- If your hamstrings are tight or if there is no blank wall, then swing your legs up onto a couch or chair.
- If your upper back is stiff or if, when you lie on your back, your head "hangs" or your chin pushes up toward the ceiling, then put a folded blanket under your head, just enough to make your head level with your heart and to bring ease to your neck.
- If you want a stronger inversion, which can promote more immediate or deeper results, then elevate your hips with a folded blanket or two. (*Note:* When you are having your menstrual cycle, don't choose to elevate your hips.)

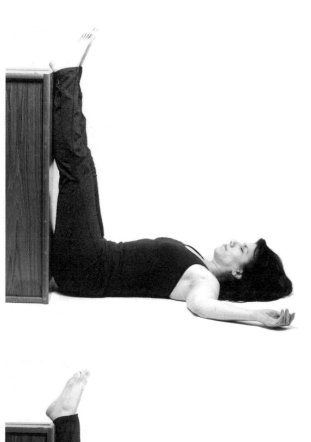

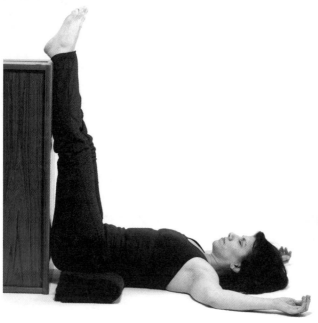

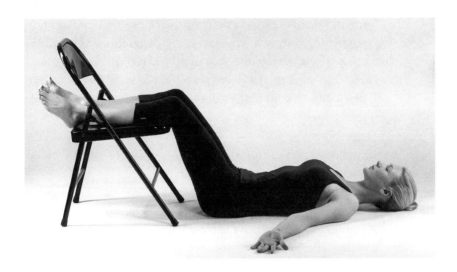

RECLINED DOUBLE-ANGLE POSE

You'll need two folded blankets and two blocks (or substitute props).

Fold the two blankets and lay them lengthwise down your yoga mat (or on the floor).

Position yourself in front of the blankets, so that when you lie back, your lumbar curve is supported by the edge of the blankets.

Curl the top blanket to support the weight of your head in such a manner that your head is slightly higher than your heart, and your gaze is down toward your heart.

Next, bring the soles of your feet together and open your knees out to the side, creating the double angles of your legs.

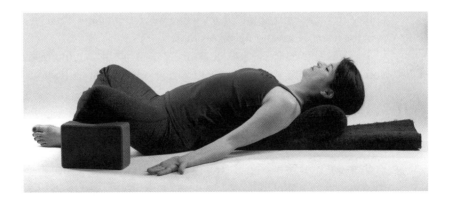

Support your knees with the yoga blocks so that you are not experiencing an inner thigh stretch. We want as few distractions as possible in this pose because it is meant to restore your mind and reduce body tension, rather than to stretch the inner thighs (there are other poses for that!).

Open your arms out to the sides with your palms facing up and your shoulders rolled open.

Suggestions:

- If your arms don't comfortably reach the floor, then try a folded bath towel under each arm.
- If your lower back hurts in this pose, then use only one lengthwise blanket under your spine.
- If your knees don't reach the blocks, then bring them closer to your pelvis, and prop them on an angle so they better support you.

PSYCHOLOGICAL RESILIENCE: RESTRAINT AND SELF-EMPATHY

Restraint is like the banks of a river, channeling its currents toward the ocean. Without healthy riverbanks, a river's energy gets dissipated or runs off into floodplains, where it never reaches the ocean. We do this to ourselves now in the form of broken promises, manipulative self-talk, conniving plans, and bargaining. Thus, one of the first restraints I'm going to suggest is to *stop* thinking these thoughts. *Stop* entertaining, trying to understand, or believing in these thoughts. Restrain your unhelpful thinking and you will have far more energy to channel toward the goal of your freedom from disordered eating patterns. Remember that one of the ways I define resilience is your "bounce-back-ability." It is easier to bounce back when we stop pushing ourselves down. This is at the heart of psychological resilience.

It is possible to free yourself from the tangle of thought clusters that keep you engaged with your disordered eating patterns. Start by becoming aware that every time you bargain with yourself for eating a certain food, every time you generate a new scheme for your weight-loss or weight-control plan, every time you "deceive yourself" again, every time you promise and then don't follow through, every time you scold yourself with an inner voice tone of shame, even every time you have a clear, wise, and skillful idea that would be useful for you but you don't allow it to come to fruition, you're setting yourself up for greater disappointment, which you register as frustration or bafflement toward yourself.

Often, we don't even realize we are playing these broadcasts. In part, this is because the way that we think about food, weight, reward, and deprivation is also very culturally driven. Our culture oozes with these broadcasts in advertising, on food packages, in the media, and in our language with each other. It is like elevator or department store music heard in the background din and mentally absorbed without our conscious knowing.

Yet we do have some control over our agreement to indulge these thoughts. Imagine it like this: cars have stereos in them, and the stereos can be programmed to go to favorite listening stations. Very often, people don't turn the stereo on and off; it's simply on all the time. Frequently, it is also playing the same station day after day. In fact, when you turn off the car at night and turn it back on in the morning, it, on its own, has not changed stations. So it will just broadcast again from your favorite station. Similarly, your mind is producing thought broadcasts all the time. You've tuned in to a few favorite stations; yet your addiction mind is the most magnetic. It pulls you to it again and again. And every time you play it, its frequency gets stronger, both in terms of its ability to keep sending signals and in the ferocity with which the messages are transmitted. (We all know how it is to get a song or even a refrain stuck in our head.)

This mental broadcast station produces the countless self-deflating pinpricks in your vitality and is profoundly hindering your resilience. Because of its impact on your mind, and thus your body, experienced as body-mind symptoms like mental restlessness, physical discomfort, fatigue, or emotional unsteadiness, this broadcast station also prevents you from establishing consistent physical sobriety, because you'll keep your particular cocktail of addiction biochemistry looping through your system. Earlier, I said recovery is going to require you to think differently. But how? Two ways: First, we start by tuning the addiction thought clusters out. Second, we shift our inner voice tone to self-empathy.

Empathy (n.):

Empathy is the capacity to recognize emotions that are being experienced by another sentient or fictional being . . . an empathic interaction involves a person communicating an accurate recognition of the significance of another person's ongoing intentional actions, associated emotional states, and personal characteristics in a manner that the recognized person can tolerate. Recognitions that are both accurate and tolerable are central features of empathy.

The human ability to recognize the bodily feelings of another is related to one's imitative capacities and seems to be grounded in an innate capacity to associate the bodily movements and facial expressions one sees in another with the proprioceptive feelings of producing those corresponding movements or expressions oneself. Humans seem to make the same immediate connection between the tone of voice and other vocal expressions and inner feeling.

— *Wikipedia*

Self-Empathy (n.):

1. Our ability to empathize with ourselves when we awaken to uncomfortable feelings such as vulnerability, fear, excitement, confidence, trepidation, or contentment. 2. An overarching quality of inner voice tone and body language that exudes tenderness, care, and compassion toward ourselves. 3. The opposite of shaming voice tone.

— *Sarahjoy*

We must staunchly, even ferociously, disagree with the broadcasts of our addiction and shame stations. We must courageously disagree with the messages that say that our value in life is based on our weight, or that our worth is connected to the size of our thighs, or that our competency is measured by our ability to stick with a life-crushing diet. On behalf of women everywhere (and all those who are impacted by the diet and exercise industries that feed us this insidious elevator music), we must stand up against this thinking.

One of the challenges we'll face, however, is the fear of standing alone, stepping out of the tribal thinking. We risk an element of alienation. Remember how much the human organism is programmed to fear alienation and yearn for belonging? Shame will try to sneak in there and seduce us back to the cultural agreement — to stay engaged with the language, the rituals, and the costs, in both time and money of investing in the diet and body image industry, and also to our health.

You'll need a big dose of restraint here. Restrain yourself from the mental broadcasts of your own addiction mind. Restrain yourself from the scary stories your shame voice will tell you about this departure from our culture. Restrain yourself from the seduction of quick-fix diet schemes, conversations about or with the scale, even discussions with others about how they're going to get their diet and exercise "thing" worked out after the New Year. Restrain yourself from the fear of being left out or outcast, or simply feeling socially awkward, and know that such restraint is going to help you restore your resilience. (I recommend that you deliberately limit the people with whom you talk about your physical goals related to weight, exercise, and nutrition to trained professionals who have knowledge of disordered eating patterns.) This restraint will also give you the chance to develop a new perspective and new community; a new voice will emerge, and you will find companions on this path. And, when you go back to that "other" community, you will be able to see the pathology clearly. You will have become an agent of change.

At present, your brain chemistry should not be randomly or repeatedly exposed to these kinds of thinking, nor to the inner voice tone that takes you down.

Here's some good news: when you restrain yourself from playing these mental broadcasts, you'll have the freedom to discover other stations in your mind. You'll have room for planning a garden, awakening your creativity, or learning a new language. When you retrain yourself from the inner voice tone of shame, you'll create the space for your self-empathy voice to thrive. You'll begin to feel understood and cherished — by your own self. Just as the body has to metabolize food, our minds have to metabolize our thinking and all the messages that it takes in during the course of the day. Freeing yourself from your addiction mind and shame-based mental broadcasts produces a big increase in your brain space and the potential for your 360-degree life!

YOGA MINDFULNESS MOMENT

Sound as Mindfulness (GAP)

When you don't know how else to tune out your mental broadcasts, try this proven technique:

Take a moment to connect to your breathing. You do not need to make a big adjustment to your breathing; simply use the breath to help you transition your attention. Shift from processing the words and ideas on these pages to listening exquisitely to the sounds around you. Whatever the sounds happen to be is fairly irrelevant. You will have preferences for some and aversion to others. Still, listen to the pulse of life around you expressed in sound. Notice also the silence through which the sounds are rising and passing. Lift the antennae of your mental attention from your mental broadcasts to the tangible evidence of life's symphony in the present moment: traffic, car door, birds, silence, children, laughter, barking dogs, silence, lawn mower, water trickle, honking horns, silence. It's all occurring in the broadcast of life that is larger than your personal broadcasts. Because our personal broadcasts rely heavily on thoughts and stories about the past and future, self and other, likes and dislikes, giving your exquisite attention to the symphony of life in this present moment is a felt relief to your mind. If you were hooked up to a biofeedback machine, it would register the change in you from arousal of your sympathetic nervous system back to your parasympathetic nervous system — in other words, from your stress response to your relaxation response.

This mindfulness practice is extremely portable and can be done anywhere, anytime. I recommend it promptly in moments of distress, preemptively in anticipation of distress, and in moments of despair or celebration, anxiety or joy.

❧ YOGA INQUIRY

The Lifeboat of Self-Empathy (MLNS)

Recall the Wikipedia definition of *empathy*: "the human ability to recognize the . . . feelings of another." This ability is "related to one's imitative capacities and . . . an innate capacity to associate the . . . facial expressions one sees in another with the proprioceptive feelings of producing those corresponding . . . expressions oneself. Humans . . . make the same immediate connection between the tone of voice and other vocal expressions." Understanding this is vital to having clear perspective about how you developed your facial patterns and voice tone when your shame is activated. This understanding is also essential for developing new facial and voice-tone responses to yourself based in self-empathy, not self-scolding.

Reflect on the unkind facial and voice-tone expressions of others that you have seen or heard when shame is present. Know that those expressions come with the countless firing of synapses flooding empathy out of their brain space.

Reflect on the facial and voice-tone expressions you encountered in earlier life, particularly when you were still developing your facial and voice-tone expressions through your imitative capacity. Now visualize what your facial and voice-tone expressions are toward yourself when you look in the mirror and succumb to shame's influence. Know that the ferocity of shame's broadcast floods empathy out of your brain space.

Imagine a durable, unsinkable lifeboat in which your self-empathy voice is carried. Imagine it bobbing down the riverbed amid shame's urge to flood you. As you catch sight of it, listen for the sound of the voice tone that reflects your self-empathy. Quite likely it has some of the following characteristics:

- tenderness (toward your pain)
- encouragement (for your courage)
- perspective (on how you got to where you are today and to where you are growing)
- kindness (toward your efforts)
- confidence (in your ability)
- protectiveness (of your recovery)

Now visualize yourself being able to hear the voice tone of self-empathy calling to you to climb aboard its lifeboat whenever shame threatens you. (When you aren't yet able to feel you deserve the whole lifeboat, self-empathy tosses you a life vest.) Visualize yourself climbing aboard: What color and shape is your lifeboat? What does it have on board with it? Is there a person (or persons) in your life, a pet, a stuffed animal, or a role model (even one you haven't met but would like to) in your lifeboat? These are the figures whose voice tone, facial expressions, eyes, ears, and hearts call to you with tenderness, perspective, and kindness. These are the voice tones and facial expressions that you will want to imitate in creating your self-empathy voice tone and facial expressions. These beings are your protectors against shame. (If you have no one to visualize in your lifeboat, put me in there for now; and as your recovery goes forward add more empathic voices, more eyes, ears, hearts, and hands.)

As you practice staying aboard the lifeboat of self-empathy, you will know with greater and greater strength that self-empathy will not allow you to be tossed overboard into shame's flood.

✢ Psychological and Physiological Resilience

Resilience is best understood as a process. It is often mistakenly assumed to be a trait of the individual, an idea more typically referred to as "resiliency." Most research now shows that resilience is the result of individuals being able to interact with their environments and *the processes that either promote well-being or that protect them against the overwhelming influence of risk factors.* These processes can be individual coping strategies, or they may be helped along by strong families, schools, communities, and social policies that make resilience more likely to occur. In this sense, *"resilience" occurs when there are cumulative "protective factors."* These factors are likely to play a more and more important role the greater the individual's exposure to cumulative risk factors. [*emphasis added*]

— *Wikipedia*

PHYSIOLOGICAL RESILIENCE: REDUCING RISK, PROMOTING VITALITY

For this section of our discussion, let's think of restraint in two ways: as preventing a destructive action (reducing your risk factors), the way a parent restrains a child from walking into a traffic intersection, and as providing protection (promoting your protective factors), the way a mother bear fiercely protects her cubs. She's programmed for this protective instinct at a time in their lives when they are unable to provide full protection to themselves. In this same regard, your wiser mind needs to fervently protect you from your addiction mind. Your wiser mind is the part of you that instinctively knows how to care for yourself. It is kind, nonjudgmental, clear, and discerning. It is capable of self-empathizing. (In the practice of yoga, you will often glimpse this wiser mind in the deep rest that follows savasana, in the moments where you glimpse clarity and love, and in the quietude of a grounded meditation.) Your wiser mind will need to intervene on food choices as well as on the habits that drain your vitality, squander critical resources, or generate symptom after symptom, keeping you in that endless cycle of symptom management that is neither sober nor resilient. Your wiser mind will be your resource for knowing when to protect you from your risk factors (such as reading material, TV programs, media influences, and certain social settings) during the earliest periods of your recovery.

A Personal Journey of Getting Sober: Reducing Risk, Promoting Vitality

As I became aware that I had a problem and that there was a world that was "clean and sober," I had an initial reaction of outrage that the very thing I struggled with the most could not be addressed in black-and-white terms. I was annoyed that "those other people" could quit smoking, quit gambling, or quit drugs, but what I had to do required me to interact with the source of my pain — food — every day. Of course I know now that it is incredibly difficult work to overcome any addiction. Yet, back then, my anger fueled my isolation and my sense of separateness from those who had "made it out."

Today I define sobriety as the restraint of coping mechanisms that dis-regulate the mind, body, and heart. These may include any substance, activity, thought, or behavior (reduce risk factors). Sobriety also provides a tremendous gift: that we learn to cherish our vitality (promote protective factors) as expressed in our body, mind, and heart.

In my process toward sobriety, there were food categories that had to be off-limits. I stayed away from bakeries, ice cream shops, and the cookie aisle in the grocery store. I could not recover my life while dis-regulated by sugar. Entering into relationship with even the smallest dose of those substances often led to painful outcomes. In fact, entering into relationship with thoughts about those foods was also problematic, because those thoughts usually included black-and-white, all-or-nothing thinking that led to distractedness, food anxiety, bingeing, and then self-hatred. So in my earliest efforts at honest sobriety, I chose not to eat sugar, not to place myself in situations where I would have ready access to certain foods (for instance, staying away from an art opening loaded with dessert buffets), and not to entertain thoughts about these foods. I chose this one day at a time. And, as sugar had previously been a reward substance for me, I had to find other ways to acknowledge and reward myself. One of the biggest things that worked for me was a hot bath. This was helpful as well because I was not willing to eat in the bathtub, nor could I compulsively exercise in there! I took a lot of hot baths in the early days of my recovery! Looking back over my life, it seems fitting that I would one day live at a hot springs retreat center and that now I have a hot tub outside my bedroom door.

Today, my relationship to food is completely wide open. I don't have food plans. I don't diet. I don't have off-limits foods. I don't white-knuckle my way past anything. I don't regret food choices or meals eaten. I don't have grocery store, restaurant, or dinner party anxiety. My weight doesn't fluctuate wildly. My thoughts are not consumed by food, body size, or self-criticism. My voice tone is steeped in self-empathy, encouragement, and positive self-regard.

During my years of struggle, this possibility was quite remote. I thought recovery would be the constant vigilance of my "good days," the days when I ate well, according to whatever my current regimen was. That constant vigilance appeared to be the only option out of my "bad days," days when I would eat compulsively, make poor food choices and regret it, fall into despairing self-hatred, or not be able to get out of bed. After a string of bad days I would always think, "I just need to work harder at this." And I would forge on in a measure of left-brain vigilance against food, confusedly trying to restrain the part of me that took over and went sliding into those bad days. Because constant vigilance also looked exhausting, undoable, institutional, and isolating, I had a very hard time convincing myself that that was a way I wanted to live. As such, with that thinking, I had a hard time gaining any ground at all in my sobriety. I kept hiking, but always below tree line. I knew what I was doing wasn't good for me. And I knew what good was supposed to look like.

Once I defined sobriety in manageable terms and set out accomplishing it one day at a time, I started feeling hopeful that recovery might be something I could achieve. And once I paired my commitment to sobriety with the practice of yoga and meditation (right-brain activities), I was able to conceive of my life being something much more remarkable than I had ever imagined. This new life, which I envisioned in my early recovery, would not be remarkable by our Western standards of wealth, status, or achievement. What would be remarkable about it would be an enormous freedom from shame, self-hatred, isolation, perfectionism, and the demands of constantly recovering from or trying to prevent food episodes. Enormous freedom. That possibility magnetically pulled me forward in every yoga pose. And yoga consistently fed my commitment to my physical sobriety as well.

One of the reasons that constant vigilance wasn't going to work for me was that it was overwhelmingly food-centered. I was battling with food as the enemy, rather than focusing on protecting my vitality. I was battling shame, rather than restoring my mental capacity to think clearly. I was battling a scale for results, rather than noting my ability to care for myself as a measure of success. At the time, I truly had no idea how exhausting and isolating this battle was to my entire being. I was very much alone in forging my path out of this cycle.

But like you, I very much wanted to be free of the pain I was in. And I was willing to stand up against my mental broadcasts and our culturally driven food- and body-based broadcasts, even if it meant standing more alone in our cultural milieu. I was willing to be ferocious against my own shame and to disavow its messages, even if only out of a blind, bold instinct. I was willing to tolerate healthy food-related restraint (i.e., sugar, refined carbohydrates) as a pathway to restore my faith in myself (a brain not under the influence of certain foods does function better!).

Little did I know it would be such a windfall in terms of also restoring my resilience, my confidence, my ability to love and nurture myself, and my courage to forge a 360-degree life that includes wider and wider circles of capacity.

Earlier, I defined sobriety as the restraint of coping mechanisms that disregulate your body, mind, and heart. Because people use coping mechanisms to regulate, attempt to manage that which feels unmanageable, soothe that which is uncomfortable (or painful or unbearable), and balance that which is out of balance, if we simply take away a coping mechanism without a suitable replacement for it, we'll be taking away protective mechanisms (albeit unhealthy ones). Self-nurturance — because it is based in love, not shame — helps us increase loving, attuned self-care to the point that it overwhelms self-harming or self-loathing. That is truly protective. To develop resilience, we increase our ability to deliver essential support and nurturance to our body. When we engage in this support and nurturance to ourselves in greater proportion than we engage in our unhealthy coping mechanisms, we overwhelm our risk factors with protective measures. Our essential life skills sound panel becomes balanced, clear, and strong.

PHYSIOLOGICAL RESILIENCE: ENGAGING THE FOUR ESSENTIAL LIFE SKILLS

Above we talked about psychological risk factors to resilience, including fear of isolation, shame, and culturally driven mental broadcasts. There are also physiological risk factors to our resilience, such as being overtired, overscheduled, overstressed, undernourished, or mentally or physically depleted. To build our physiological resilience, we return to the four essential life skills.

Getting in the GAP: Your Body Dashboard

In chapter 5 we discussed "Unearthing Faith: Creating Personal Buoyancy through Self-Accountability" and in chapter 4, the "Reasonable Guidelines for Respecting Your Body Intelligence and Nourishing Your Life Vitality." Now let's synthesize those previous suggestions into an easy-to-remember metaphor: dashboarding. Consider it like this: your car has a dashboard with a series of lights and signals. You know when your car is low on fuel, overheating, in cruise control mode, and a host of other functions. With my Prius I have a specific screen that tells me when I am using fuel and when I am using the battery. Your body has a dashboard, a fuel tank, and a battery, too. Your ability to read your dashboard signals, to know when to fill your fuel tank, and to be aware when you are relying on your battery have been confused by yo-yo dieting, bingeing, purging, restricting, and over- or underexercise regimens that were not in harmony with the demands of a physical body. You, like millions of others, are too practiced at not reading your body's dashboard, not filling your fuel tank, and ignoring your battery (and you live in a culture that reinforces this habit).

Your physical body, called the *annamayakosha* in yoga, is your muscles, bones, organs, and connective tissue. Your physical body both affects and is the expression of your vitality, or your "energy body," called the *pranamayakosha*, which includes your respiration, circulation, and innervation, and your mind, called the *mannamayakosha*, which includes your perceptions, reactions, and emotions. It's a two-way conversation, much like between you and your car. Your dashboard tells you the speed you are driving and dutifully reflects the results of your stepping on the accelerator or the brake. Your car has mechanisms for managing the heating and cooling systems, and if there is a problem, you are alerted by signals on your dashboard.

Likewise, your body signals you constantly. Fortunately, it has a host of preprogrammed, intelligent functions that manage your internal environment without your conscious knowing. There are millions of small adjustments your body's intelligence makes to regulate your body temperature, protect your brain, and manage your blood pressure for simple tasks such as standing from sitting, climbing hills, taking a hot shower, or riding in a car. Luckily for you, you don't have to keep track of all of this! You are going to greatly benefit, however, from keeping track of just a few critical areas that are under your direct control: hydration, rest, fresh air, movement, nourishment, and elimination (these were all mentioned in "Reasonable Guidelines for Respecting Your Body Intelligence and Nourishing Your Life Vitality" on p. 136).

To fill your gas tank, and boost your confidence and brain function, you'll need the basics: enough water, enough rest, enough fresh air, balanced movement or exercise, balanced blood sugar and general nourishment, and timely elimination. (Reflect back on Maslow's hierarchy of needs and our discussion on self-accountability.) It is shocking to realize how many times we postpone a trip to the bathroom to relieve our bladder because of an e-mail marathon. Or we don't get ourselves a glass of water because we're working on something else. Our body and brain will function much better when we tend to these essentials! Incorporating these essentials into your daily life will markedly increase your optimism about your recovery. It will require you to protect your vitality and to show up for yourself, fervently at times. It will require you to know how to read your dashboard!

YOGA INQUIRY

Dashboarding as a Recovery Skill (GAP)

Dashboarding means reading your dashboard, then wisely and proactively responding. This is different from driving a car and waiting for the dashboard light to come on to signal us. In recovery, checking our dashboard is a preemptive act of mindfulness. As you learn the art of this, it takes less than one minute. In the beginning, it may take more time. Much like learning any new skill, every time you work with the skill, you build its efficiency and effectiveness.

Using the voice tone of self-empathy, an overarching quality of inner voice tone that exudes tenderness and care, spend four deep breaths on each of your seven dashboard cues: rest, thirst, fresh air, movement, nourishment, elimination, and right-brain activities.

- How rested do you feel? Have you had a sufficient amount of rest for the task at hand? Is what you are engaged in causing fatigue? (Sometimes when our brains are learning new things, paradigm-shifting things, it can get fatigued like muscles doing a new physical activity. If we don't prioritize rest, we're more likely to fall back on familiar behaviors.)
- Are you thirsty? How thirsty? Have you been hydrating today?

- Have you had fresh air on your face today? Is your body or mind asking for a few moments in nature?
- Is your body asking you to do some movement or raise your heart rate (even for sixty seconds)?
- Does your brain need nutrition? Are you having any blood sugar fluctuations? What has your hunger-to-satiation spectrum been like today?
- Does your bladder need to be emptied? Are you postponing a trip to the bathroom to read this paragraph, write an e-mail, or have a conversation?
- Additionally, have you laughed or cried today?
- Have you explored a right-brain activity today?

Now that you've checked the signals on your dashboard, you have the life-sustaining responsibility of responding. Millions of people postpone the basic needs of their physical body, chronically, constantly, proudly. But you are going to be an agent of change in this regard. Your body should not be tolerating postponement, not at this juncture in your recovery. Every time your body gives you a signal and you are able to wisely respond, you're promoting your protective factors while simultaneously preventing and reducing your risk factors. This is not just a mathematical breakthrough. It is the breakthrough of opportunity over danger. Each signal is an opportunity to practice promoting resilience and increasing your self-empathy.

- If you discover that you are tired and need more rest, take savasana for five minutes.
- If you discover that your body is thirsty, promptly get some water.
- If you realize your body is craving fresh air, step outdoors for a minute, five minutes, or take direction from your self-accountability list (p. 153), and go for twenty minutes of mindful time outdoors with the air against your skin.
- If you discover that you haven't raised your heart rate to adjust your physiology today, try a quick burst of activity: climb a flight of stairs dynamically, do some jumping jacks, or use the breath of joy (p. 119) or saying *no* to say *yes* (p. 78) exercises. Raising your heart rate for twenty minutes is still a priority, but achievable (brief, portable, and effective) interventions are also important.
- If you discover that your blood sugar is low, promptly address this with healthy protein in a reasonable portion.
- If you realize that you have to use the bathroom, promptly do so.
- If you realize that you haven't laughed or cried today, create a way to do one or the other. This part of your dashboard should not be overlooked.

You can practice and promote laughing and crying. One of the ways that I teach students to do this is by using YouTube videos that stir us about the poignancy and joy of the human spirit. (Visit www.sarahjoyyoga.com for a list of videos my students have recommended.)

Getting Comfortable Feeling Uncomfortable: Adjusting Your Physiology (GCFU)

Far too often, our self-medicating, food-driven, compulsive-thinking issues could be overcome if we proactively take a few moments of dashboarding to get current with ourselves. There is a very real physiological component to our urges for behaviors as well as certain thought clusters. We're more vulnerable when we're tired, dehydrated, overly hungry, suffering a blood sugar crash, or carrying pent-up physical energy that brews into restlessness, lethargy, anxiety, or depression. These are the physiological risks to sobriety. At this stage of your recovery, addressing these risks is essential.

We could posit that from the beginning, our now-compulsive behaviors were simply efforts to shift our physiology from something uncomfortable, such as anxiety, to something more comfortable or manageable, such as numbness. With the agency we had when we were very young, food and the restriction of food were both available tools, along with detaching or dissociating from our body, freezing emotions, bottling up anger, turning to TV or media to numb ourselves, being perfectionistic, engaging in cleanliness rituals, and weighing and evaluating ourselves. One of the unfortunate outcomes is that these early life strategies worked to get us out of pain in such a way that we kept using them at the expense of developing new skills, developing a more intimate and loving relationship to our body, and learning to understand how our thoughts and feelings are looped into and affecting our physiology. When addictive behavior is practiced enough, we also lose our leadership over our own behavior. We may have been looking to control our physiological or mental experiences of distress, but now the behaviors that once worked have control over us. This is one way to define the phenomenon: "We can't stop it. It has become more powerful than we are."

Recovery poses a new challenge in getting comfortable feeling uncomfortable: feeling the "uncomfortable" in getting quiet, or in experiencing contentment, hope, or joy. I don't want you to derail yourself when you're feeling good or hopeful any more than when you're feeling bad. The mind-body intervention tools below are for adjusting your physiology in support of you regaining some leadership over that physiology.

YOGA MINDFULNESS MOMENT
Mind-Body Interventions (GCFU)

I recommend the following tactile, sensory-based, mind-body interventions for shifting your physiology and coming back to the open sky of your mind. The open sky of your mind can be discovered as you might find the tiny sky inside the snow globe, which becomes clear of snowstorms after being shaken and set back on the counter. These exercises are designed to promote a shift in your physiology that can then settle itself down, just like your snow globe. When you explore each of these exercises, use them as opportunities to promote the voice tone of self-empathy and prevent the voice tone of self-rejection or shame. Recovery requires you to feel uncomfortable things. It's courageous to do so. You deserve the support of your own empathy while experiencing vulnerability, fear, excitement, and beyond!

HOT TEA MUG

Fill a tea mug halfway with hot water. Depending on the mug you have chosen, it may be too hot to hold with full palms. Likely, the upper part of the mug will be cooler than the bottom. Hold it with both hands in a manner that is not going to be too hot to tolerate. Set your mind to paying attention to the temperature and texture of the tea mug. Specifically, observe how immediately your hands respond to the temperature of the cup, as well as how they experience the different temperatures of the upper part, the handle, and the bottom part of the mug. Slowly the cup will cool down and you will be able to hold it without it being too hot. Be attentive enough to notice this incremental and intimate experience. Observe how your mind can become more still as the mug becomes not just easier to hold but also comforting to hold. If it helps your mind to stay fresh, try lifting one finger or hand off the mug and then replacing it anew. Recognize the changing temperature of the finger as it moves away from and back to the mug.

Texture as Teacher

Pick an object that has a specific texture, like a stone, a particular scarf, or a smooth or bumpy object. Bring your attention to the texture as your hands experience it without moving them. Then slowly move your hands around the object with the explicit intention to *feel* the texture, to immerse your mind in the exquisite tactile experience. Do not let your mind wander away from the texture. However, when it does (it might!), bring it back to the exquisite experience of texture again.

Hot and Cold

A hot shower followed by a cold shower is a tremendous opportunity to shift your physiology, rapidly. Take a five-minute hot shower, followed by thirty seconds of a cold shower. Repeat two or three times, as needed, finishing with cold. This exercise provides a physiological rush, and shakes your mind out of restless ruminations or dissociations back into the here and now.

If you cannot do an entire shower, try the same technique with hot and cold water on your hands, or a warm to hot washcloth on your face, followed by cold splashes of water.

Environmental Awareness

Become keenly aware of your physical environment and practice narrowing the aperture of what you think about and to what you give your attention. When thought threatens to overwhelm your mind, fix it on counting the number of petals on a tulip, how many blossoms are waiting to open in a columbine, or how many floorboards are between you and the door to the room. If there is a particular sound in your environment, give your focus to the nuances hidden within the sound. (See the exercise Sound as Mindfulness on p. 189.)

Shaking Off Cobwebs

As you may occasionally feel you have cobwebs in your brain (mental fogginess, old habits haunting your thinking), learning to shake off the cobwebs is very freeing. Stand up and vigorously swing your arms simultaneously from front to back and back to front, repeatedly. With each vigorous swing of the arms back, make your hands into fists. With each swing, exhale through your nose, swing your arms forward, and spread your fingers wide. Inhale strongly

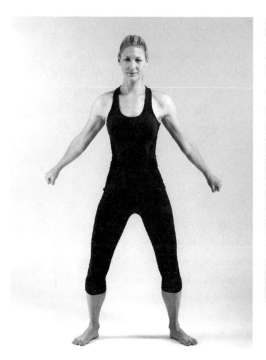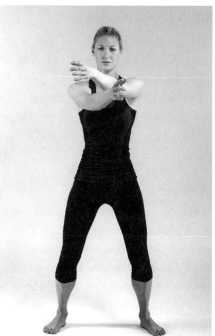

through your nose. Do this rhythmically for a minimum of one minute. Then let your arms swing and slow down to stillness. Take a deep, long inhalation through your nose and completely exhale out your nose. Notice any greater capacity in your lungs, or a sense of space in your mind or heart. Repeat as needed.

RAISED HEART RATE

Raising your heart rate for a few minutes (or moments) is powerfully effective in shifting your mind-body physiology. In this exercise, something simple, doable, and portable works best. Jumping rope or doing jumping jacks are probably familiar options. You can also try a simple technique of bouncing up and down. Small rhythmic bounces can help shift energy, and can become larger bounces if you feel safe doing so. Alternatively, a quick walk up a steep hill is wonderful. (And gets some air against your skin!)

PRESSURE-SHIFTING YOGA POSES

Yoga practices include inversions, which powerfully shift the pressure systems of the body. (We can think of these as being like weather pressure systems.)

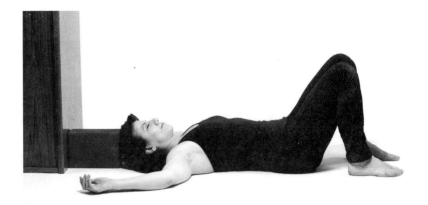

Yet we're not all meant to do inversions, especially those who are new to the practice of yoga. Here are some "pseudo-inversions" that also create a pressure system change in the body-mind-psyche.

- Reclined headstand: Put a yoga block at the baseboard of a wall. Lie down with your knees bent and position the crown of your skull against the block. Place your arms out to the side or in cactus pose. Bring the small of your back down to the floor. Pressing with your feet, gradually increase the pressure of your head into the block, while maintaining some length in your neck. Breathe softly into the belly without urgency. Maintain this for one or two minutes. Upon releasing, simply relax your efforts and lie still. Observe the effects on your mind and body.

- Seated shoulderstand breathing: Sit on the edge of a chair. Place your hands on the sides of the chair, higher up if your shoulders are more flexible. Lift your chest and bring your chin down toward your throat. While keeping the shoulders rolled open, inhale and exhale slowly and deeply using your diaphragm (you should feel your belly expanding and contracting). Inhale through your nose; exhale through pursed lips (to slow down the exhale and make it longer than your inhale). Put a slight pause at the top of inhales and bottom of exhales. Do this for one or two minutes with the intention of slowing down your breathing to help slow down your mind. When you finish, rest your hands in your lap and allow your breathing to return to resting. Observe the effects on your mind and body.

- Also recommended: pressure-release-valve breathing (p. 119) and the legs-up-the-wall pose (p. 183).

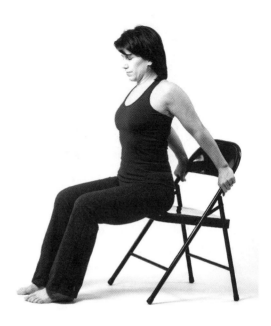

These practices also become more powerful when done regularly. Just like disordered eating behaviors became more powerful, more automatic, and more seductive with practice (repetition), these yoga exercises also become more automatic, more natural, and more capable of pulling you through a stormy moment in your recovery. Think of it like this: when you are distressed, somehow, sneakily, the thought of a certain food might arise, and then the thought of how and when you will have that food. Even if you can't get to the food promptly, the thought that you can have it later brings on enough ease to bear the moment. You're in a meeting. You're feeling [bored, exposed, unprepared, overwhelmed, confused, unimportant], and an image of a chocolate chip cookie comes to mind. You might battle it for a moment or two, but your mind has already produced the image and suggested the possibility. Once you think of it and recognize that you could have the cookie later — in fact, that you *will* have the cookie later — you experience just enough ease to bear the uncomfortable feeling and get through the meeting.

What if this could happen instead: you're in the meeting, the same scenario is unfolding, and your mind produces the image of the "shaking off cobwebs" or "hot and cold" exercises as tools to work out the physiological rush of the body-mind "storm" and allow you to experience your self-empathy voice tone, the one that acknowledges the courage, conviction, and confidence you're developing?

Moving from Love, not Shame: Ending the Isolation (MLNS)

One of the painful things about disordered eating patterns is the way they isolate us. I noted earlier that disordered eating has a unique pain in its ability to cause this isolation; it is not a commonly practiced thing in "groups." People at happy hour are using a socially acceptable activity with a socially acceptable substance to shift their mental and physiological state. My use of this example isn't to implicate them in having an alcohol problem per se, but to note that alcohol is a substance, and social drinking is a behavior, that carries less shame and more cultural acceptance. (Certainly, people who identify as having a problem with alcohol experience shame.) For those of us struggling with disordered eating behavior, we engage in these activities clandestinely rather than in groups. In fact, sometimes spouses or people who live with us don't even know the disordered behavior is happening. There has been an element of secrecy and isolation in the way we move through our robotic, alien-invader rituals. This isolation makes us more vulnerable to shame, as it tells us how bad we are and how we are the only ones struggling like this. Yet another way that we promote painful isolation is through the lack of kindheartedness toward ourselves. We are pushed out of the realm of our own empathy and create the conditions of self-abandonment.

Ending the isolation is absolutely critical in recovery from disordered eating patterns. We need to know that we don't have to do the difficult and often scary things all by ourselves; we don't need to keep hiding, and we don't need to be isolated. We can have empathy toward ourselves — and at the same time we need to know that our recovery matters to someone else.

Before I teach you the process of ending the isolation, let me acknowledge something about kindheartedness and self-empathy. Countless women have reported to me a belief that if they were to be kindhearted toward themselves they would never get better. If they were to express self-empathy, they would become lazy slugs, not eating better, not exercising better, not doing any of the things they know they are supposed to be doing, or not doing the things they would need to do to make up for the bad things they are doing. This is a myth. I promise you. You have already experienced this; you have not gotten any better by being mean to yourself. By being coldhearted or condescending, you have not made any lasting improvements. Nonetheless, women insist, "If I don't control myself, I will lose control." "If I don't do this [personal behavior related to controlling their weight], I will get fat." And so on.

This is simply not a useful or considerate way to look at this. It is one-sided (implies that you need to be "controlled"), unfair (points the finger at the part of you that is "out of control"), ineffective (you already know this one), narrow-minded (assumes something about your basic nature that you think is the way you will always be), and painfully isolating. The process of recovery, of living your 360-degree life, is a holistic undertaking. The thought process of "I need to control myself" assumes there is only one intervention. And, we all know by now, that intervention hasn't been working.

In all of the groups, workshops, and retreats I have ever facilitated for women with disordered eating patterns, one thing I can always count on is that women will say one or more of the following:

"I thought it was just me. I can't believe it's not."
"I thought I was the only one who acted crazy like this. It is such a relief to know I am not crazy, and that I am not alone."
"You just perfectly described me. How did you know? I thought I was the only one who struggled like that!"

In each other's company, the healing begins. Reading this book will certainly help you with your healing process. Yet it truly is essential that you build a network of support that helps you end the isolation. In isolation, your conditioned-mind thoughts will have too much power over your courageous-mind thoughts.

Proactive Steps to Take

- Join me in my online community discussions (see Resources).
- Attend a retreat or workshop.
- Read from the suggested book list, and actively visualize the community you are a part of — the community that is also reading the books you choose.
- Scan your friendship group for any one person you know who will always empathetically, respectfully, and lovingly accept and support you. If you don't have someone like that, ask me about the Attunement Network at www.sarahjoyyoga.com. The Attunement Network is a group of others committed to recovery from disordered eating patterns. Using social

media tools, such as the confidential group on my website, women connect with other women with the explicit purpose of providing empathy and support for each other, of being a lighthouse for each other when the sea is stormy.

- Interview yoga teachers to find out whether they have experience helping people with disordered eating patterns. (Please note, experience is *very* helpful. However, some yoga teachers will be able to help you even if they don't have training. They may seek out mentorship from another yoga teacher who does have experience.)
- Find a skilled therapist.

YOGA INQUIRY

Ending the Isolation: Daily Practices (MLNS)

ACKNOWLEDGMENT

The grocery clerk. The salesperson. The garbage pickup person. The delivery person. Acknowledge the often "invisible" others who cross your path during the day. You're acknowledging their coexisting presence on the planet, and the humanity in them. You don't have to say or do anything external. In fact, I don't even recommend doing so. You are just taking the time not to overlook them or take them for granted, but rather to notice them and feel your interconnected existence with them.

AUTHENTICITY

Even if you don't have someone with whom you can share your story, you can still create personal opportunities for greater authenticity. Some examples include stating your preferences, speaking up about choosing a movie or a restaurant, saying something in a meeting, stating a boundary, or verbalizing a personal preference for a shared activity. Speaking up might also include setting boundaries around time management and sharing those limits with anyone they might affect. For example, "I'd enjoy meeting you for tea. That sounds lovely. And I will need to be done with our visit by about 3 P.M. Will that work for your schedule?"

In other ways, authenticity might require getting quiet. This could include not being the one who has to speak up "all the time." It could include listening and not offering advice, not engaging in reflexive problem-solving, not engaging in reflexive gossiping, or not making unfocused chatter "about nothing."

KINDHEARTEDNESS

Kindhearted gestures toward yourself are capable of creating radical shifts in your self-esteem.

- Buy yourself flowers. Set up several small vases in your living environment so that you'll be aware of them throughout your house. Tend to those flowers so they don't go bad too soon!
- Light a candle in your home or at your desk as a reminder of your commitment to your recovery.
- Wear a special ring that symbolizes your commitment to your recovery.
- Walk the long way home from the bus stop and enjoy the luxury of time to stroll with yourself.
- Purchase some lovely greeting cards that are blank on the inside. Write yourself messages of appreciation, courage, strength, and acknowledgment. Seal, address, and stamp the cards. Drop them in the mailbox. Open them when they arrive (don't leave them in the pile of mail that stacks up). Save the cards for repeated reading. Do this regularly and it will become a way to sustain your recovery when the shame voice kicks in!

CONNECTION

Look at the ways in which you cause yourself to feel isolated by being in relationships or social environments in which you're not alone but you are lonely. If you are in relationships or environments that aren't particularly unhealthy yet you hold yourself back from participating, and thus experience isolation, there are two practices you can start with: (1) listen intently to what others are saying and seek the common humanity between you and (2) verbalize your interest in them. This might look like asking a question about what they've been talking about ("How did you choose to vacation in Assisi?" "How did you get interested in bowling?"), saying something that indicates your interest ("That's interesting. Would you be willing to tell me more about that?"), or reflecting back what you heard them say ("It sounds like you really enjoyed the graduation ceremony.").

If you must be in relationships or environments that are unhealthy for you (a job, a relative, a coworker), learn to actively listen to the other humans and hear their humanity, even in the ways in which it might be troubled, anxious, or immature. Listening is a way to pull yourself out of your disconnect habit. What I recommend you connect to in these "others" is their humanity, not their personality. Listen with an ear toward tenderness for their humanity. Our own foibles may be more comfortable to us, yet all human foibles can be doorways to compassion.

Still, we must wisely choose whom we rely on in ending our isolation. Shame is made more powerful by our isolation, but it is also made more powerful when we choose people who can't understand, support, or encourage us. Some relationships or environments will not be ones in which you can practice. That doesn't mean that you ought not practice.

Personal Buoyancy: Your Life Vitality (PB)

Just as the sun is at the center of our planet's orbit, so, too, at the source of our vitality is a radiant force yoga calls *ananda*. Recovery is the process of reconnecting to this vital source. Much like the vitality our plants gain when we provide water to our garden, when we are hooked up to this source of radiant vitality, we'll experience much greater ease and more successful outcomes. For example, to most effectively and easily water a garden, you need a well-functioning system for getting the water to the plants. If your hose isn't hooked up to the water source, has leaks in it, or isn't pointing in the right direction, your garden will not flourish. And trying to water your garden under those conditions will be wasteful, requiring greater resources (it takes both more water and more time to water a garden with a hose that has holes in it), and may only partially water the plants. You, and your recovery, deserve the greatest chance at flourishing. To see to this, you must hook yourself up to the source of your vitality, prevent the chronic drains on your energy, and hone your attention and efforts in the optimal direction.

Reconnecting to the Source

The *koshas* represent the layers of our human experience physically, energetically, mentally, and spiritually. Like ripples on water, they begin from the center. At the center of the koshas is love, deep contentment, quiet joy, and belonging, called the *anandamayakosha* (the level at which we experience ananda). Intimately linked to this is the layer of our intuition, clarity,

koshas

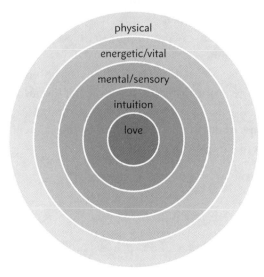

physical

energetic/vital

mental/sensory

intuition

love

Figure 6.3

and wise presence, called the *vijnanamayakosha*. Anandamayakosha is the energy that fuels our physical, mental, emotional, and vital health. When we are consistently connected to this source, we experience vibrancy, joy, contentment, and love (toward ourselves and others) in an ongoing, uninterrupted way. Most of us don't live like this, whether we have an addiction or not. We experience far more exhaustion than vibrancy, more disappointment than contentment, and more self-hatred than love. As a result, we live with skepticism or denial about the possibility that this source of vitality could be nourishing us. Yet in spite of our skepticism, even in spite of our blatant resistance or years of self-harming behavior, something goes on beating our hearts and breathing our lungs (even when we have not one ounce of awareness about it). Yoga doesn't take this for granted. Rather, it is cause for reverence toward the intelligence that circulates our blood, ripens the fruits of the trees, and brings flowers into bloom.

Most humans in today's world feel disconnected from this primordial, life-giving source. We're more connected to our technology than we are to deep presence. We're more tuned in to the news than we are to ourselves. We're more aware of the weather report than we are of our own body's reciprocity with the rhythms of nature. As a result, we see and experience a wide range of physical symptoms, such as restlessness, anxiety, depression, fatigue, or pain; lifestyle conditions, such as heart disease, obesity, chronic headaches, or addiction; and social ills, such as pettiness, gossip, grasping, aversion, and an overarching emptiness to which we numb ourselves with alcohol, food, television, or other forms of self-medication. We've become profoundly nonresilient, incapable of tolerating anything outside of our comfort zones.

One of the most poignant elements of this sad state of affairs is that we acclimate to our surroundings. The more dull life is around us, the more likely we are to acclimate to dullness as an acceptable standard. The more frenzied those around us are, the more likely we are to be magnetically pulled into such frenzy. As I said in chapter 4, your disordered eating patterns are messages from your body that something is terribly out of balance. I posit that one critical piece of news your body is trying to tell you is that acclimating to a life under this pervasive, even unquestioned, disconnection, whether it shows up as dullness, frenzy, or a combination of both, is intolerable to your deepest self. In a way, it's you trying to elbow your way out of that too-small framework for living. In order to "break out" of this framework, you'll need to repair your resilience, because you can expect a period of "not fitting in" with parts of your cultural or social norms. You will need to restore your physical vitality in order to feed your mental endurance and clarity. You'll do these things best by reconnecting, or hooking yourself back up, to the source of what yoga refers to as the "center of being," or ananda.

To water your garden, to nourish your vital life, you must hook up the hose to the water source, the source of your vitality. In yoga, that connection is made when you experience your breath in your body. When you embrace the possibility that life is breathing itself into you because you belong here and because you deserve to live with vibrancy, then you are further securing your connection to this source.

If you've internalized shame deeply enough, you may find this notion excruciating, even preposterous. You may feel that you have already demonstrated to yourself, to others, even to me, that you are outside the circle of deep belonging. Yet I have complete confidence in you and in your deep belonging—because I had to find it in myself. From the vantage point of more than twenty-five years into my recovery, I am talking to you. And I will say it again: I have complete confidence in you and in your deep belonging. I know that shame has hidden this from your own knowing and has disconnected you from the source of your vitality. I know that you can recover this. I know this as surely as I know that, without your conscious consent or direction, your fingernails are growing themselves, your lungs are breathing themselves, and your skin is feeling the surface of this book. I also know this is hard work. At times, you will need your all-out fervency to remember, to reconnect, and to take your place in the circle of belonging.

☙ YOGA MOMENT

Reconnecting to the Source of Your Vitality (PB)

Our body pulses with life force, which yoga calls *prana*. We can experience prana directly in our breathing, in our heart rate, and in the tingle of our skin when we experience temperature changes. Being awakened to this life force can be a joyful adventure! Here are three simple yoga exercises in which you can directly experience these sensations.

RECLINED MOUNTAIN POSE WITH UPWARD HANDS

Lie on your back with your legs outstretched. Reach your arms overhead and actively stretch into your fingers, thumbs, heels, and toes. Imagine you are being pulled in both directions by an outside force. As you reach actively, deepen your breath in your lower belly, inhaling and exhaling through your nose. Keep the activation of all of the muscles and bones in your limbs and open your belly to the breath by releasing any tension in the belly.

Do this for two minutes.

Then release every effort you are making and let your body lie limp in whatever position it craves. Closely observe how your body tingles, how your muscles melt after exertion, how the blood flow shifts in your limbs, and how your belly softens after your efforts. Feel your body being breathed.

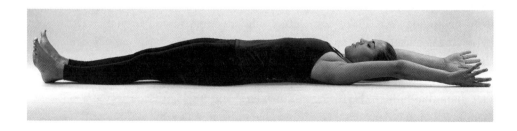

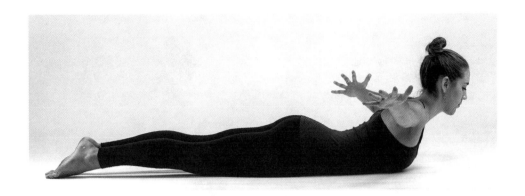

SALAMBASANA POSE

This is a belly-down backbend pose that generates strength and vitality.

Lie on your stomach with your arms outstretched in the shape of the letter T. Momentarily, center your forehead on the floor and connect to your breath. Energize your legs and root your tailbone toward the floor, which ought to lengthen your lower back. Then, with an inhale, lift your arms, chest, heart, shoulders, and head, without jutting your chin forward. When you lift, your body will need more oxygen, so deepen your inhale and be patient with your exhale. Strongly energize your arms, like the wings of a great bird, especially at the back of your shoulders. Deliberately squeeze those muscles to wake them up. You will be increasing your blood flow, body temperature, and heart rate. Try to breathe deeply but slowly.

Do this for one minute.

Then release everything completely. Make your hands into a pillow for your head as you come down out of the pose to rest. Closely observe the way the muscles on your upper back melt, notice the temperature changes in your upper back, and how your breathing rhythmically settles down. Finally, observe your heart rate slowing down as well.

BASIC LUNGE POSE

Come to your hands and knees in table pose. Then step your right foot forward between your hands, so that your chest comes down over your right thigh. Keep your fingertips on the floor, or use a set of yoga blocks to make the floor easier to reach (or any other prop that you can use to support yourself). Then straighten your left leg behind you. The best position for your front shin is 90 degrees over your ankle, from front to back and from left to right. The front

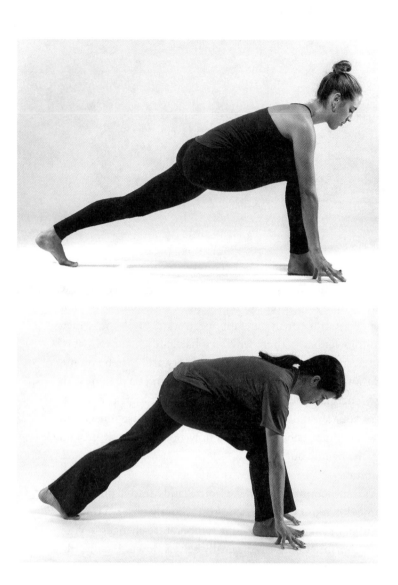

thigh can be fairly low to the floor, but not lower than horizontal. The back leg should be straight, strong, and energized. Your back heel will not reach the floor in this position. With your chest touching your thigh, you will be temporarily compressing the femoral artery.

Press your front heel down very strongly. Equally, lengthen your back leg in opposition to your front leg. Breathe deeply into your belly.

Hold the pose for one minute.

Pay very close attention when you release the pose. You will notice a temperature change in the leg, as well as a kind of tingle of aliveness. To release, step your right foot back into a push-up position, which yoga calls plank pose. (It is okay to do the plank pose with your hands on your yoga blocks, as long as the blocks are positioned in a stable manner. I have found that some blocks are thinner than others and may not provide the stability that you need.) After several moments of observing your body regulate its vital flow of blood, temperature, and heart rate, place your knees down into table pose, where you started this sequence.

Change sides and repeat.

Upright Lunge Pose

For round two, from your basic lunge pose inhale deeply. Then exhale and root your tailbone down. From there inhale and rise up to the upright lunge pose with your arms overhead. From the center of your pose, exude radiance and courage (even if you are faking it for now).

Breathe deeply into your pose for ten breath cycles. Let your mind get still even though your heart rate and breath rate are increasing.

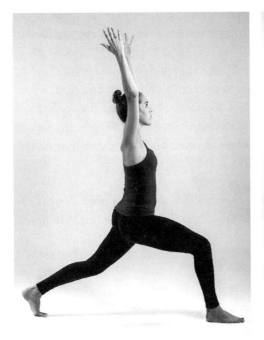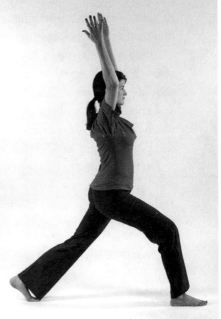

Then exhale and bow forward over your front leg to touch the floor. Step back into table pose and then do child's pose.

Repeat on the second side, reflecting in child's pose for a minute.

This four-pose "yoga set" can be accomplished in less than twelve minutes, and it makes a good preparation for meditation.

 YOGA MOMENT

The Circle of Belonging (PB)

That which grows the daffodils and sustains the rhythmic waves of the ocean also sustains, infuses, and envelops you. Although addiction has the power to make us feel terribly separate from this experience, yoga has the power to bring us back. Through the practices of yoga, we lessen the feelings of alienation and inadequacy. These poses with the breathing emphasis will help you explore this.

CHEST-OPENING POSE WITH DOOR FRAME

At the times when we feel downtrodden, contracted, lonely, angry, or frustrated, opening the chest may not feel like our first inclination. Yet recovery partly consists of our willingness to try something different, even to experiment with the opposite inclination!

Stand within an open door frame. Place your hands on the sides of the door frame, and then step through the doorway to open your chest and stretch your shoulders and arms. Breathe deeply into your belly and imagine your torso and arms like the sail of a ship. Let the breath become the wind in the sail. (If you have longer arms or more tightness in your shoulders, bend your elbows and position your hands lower on the door frame.)

Do this for one to two minutes.

When you release, do so slowly. Step backward into the open door frame again. Release your arms down by your sides and observe the tingle, temperature, and weight of your arms.

TRIANGLE POSE

This is a standing pose that stretches the legs, spine, and chest.

Take a stance, on a yoga mat or nonskid surface, with your feet about three to four feet apart (depending on your height). With your heels lined up, turn

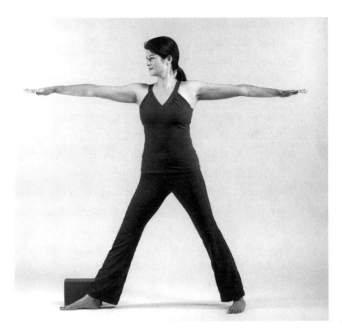

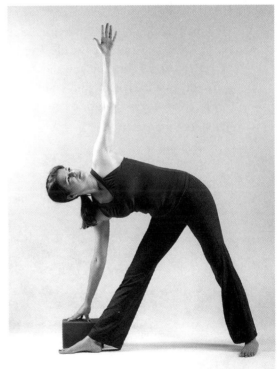

your right foot open to your right and turn your left foot slightly in. Lift your chest and spread your arms wide. Imagine a large circle of energy that encompasses you surrounding both hands, both feet, and the top of your head. Stretch out in all five directions. Then with an exhale, bend to your right sideways and slide your right hand down your right leg until your hand rests on your shin, a chair, a yoga block, or the floor, without leaning your chest forward or your hips back. Tone all the muscles of your legs and actively open your chest. Deepen your breath into your belly and lengthen again in all five directions. As you reach up, out, and down, press yourself out into that imaginary circle with the conviction of your own belonging. Even if you have to pretend, try it on. Daffodils don't hide themselves. Hummingbirds don't question their place in the sun. Fawns don't get frustrated about their newborn legs. Press yourself out into the circle of belonging to these miracles. You are one of them. You always have been. Breathe it in to every cell of your body.

Stay in the pose for one minute.

Inhale to come up out of the pose. Then repeat on the other side.

BRIDGE POSE

We'll be building on two practices from chapter 4: the inflating breath and the pressure-release-valve breath. This time our emphasis is on dissolving any perceived barrier between you and your deep sense of belonging.

Lie on your back with your knees bent.

Place your arms alongside your torso and tuck your shoulders under your upper back.

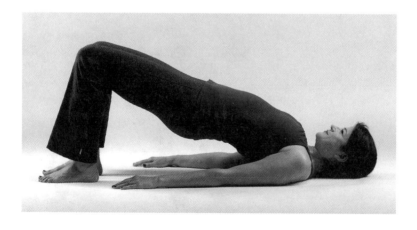

Settle your mind and recall the effects of the chest-opening pose and the triangle pose. Notice how your torso, lungs, shoulders, and heart feel. Become aware of your breathing.

When you feel ready, press down into both feet and lift your hips up to bridge pose, called so because the hips and spine form a backbend resembling a bridge. Lengthen your tailbone toward your knees and lift your heart and chest toward the sky.

Inhale very deeply from the base of your belly, up through your midtorso, and into your heart region. When you have filled your lungs to capacity, hold the breath very momentarily. You'll feel your chest expand from the inside. Imagine the pressure of the breath pressing from the inside out against any inner body tension, in your belly, ribs, chest, or heart.

Then exhale long and slow through your nose. Dissolve whatever tension you've become aware of. Imagine this dissolving away in order to reveal what is deeply, innately true beneath your accumulated stress, tension, or mental habits: you have a place of belonging here, in your body, in your life, in the circle of life itself. You always have.

Do this breath three times before releasing the pose. When you come down, pause and reflect on the tensions you dissolved and the open space this creates.

Repeat the pose three times.

Then rest while internally emphasizing your place in the family of things, as Mary Oliver has named it in her majestic poem "Wild Geese."

WILD GEESE

You do not have to be good.
You do not have to walk on your knees
For a hundred miles through the desert, repenting.
You only have to let the soft animal of your body
love what it loves.
Tell me about despair, yours, and I will tell you mine.
Meanwhile the world goes on.
Meanwhile the sun and the clear pebbles of the rain
are moving across the landscapes,
over the prairies and the deep trees,
the mountains and the rivers.

Meanwhile the wild geese, high in the clean blue air,
are heading home again.
Whoever you are, no matter how lonely,
the world offers itself to your imagination,
calls to you like the wild geese, harsh and exciting —
over and over announcing your place
in the family of things.

7

CAUSES OF SUFFERING, SOURCES OF JOY

A S WE CONTINUE THE STEPS OF SELF-STUDY, we must ask, "From where do the patterns of our mental broadcasts come? How do we think what we think? How do we shift our thinking from one level of understanding or consciousness to the next? How do we create the inner environment where self-empathy thrives over shame?"

None of us can remember learning to walk or talk. We literally have no memory of how we accomplished these ordinary human developmental experiences. That's not because we have poor memory, but rather because the developmental age and stage of our brain at the time we were learning to walk and talk wasn't set up to form and store such cognitive memories. Similarly, without having to chart a deliberate map across new terrain we went through other developmental stages, such as learning how to share (observe toddlers and you'll see them growing through this developmental stage) or being able to see an experience through the eyes of another (the sense that we disappear when we cover our own eyes in peekaboo no longer works at a certain age).

I'm using these psycho-social-biological examples because part of our brain is preprogrammed to work through such imperatives. Additionally, much of our brain and, as a result, our thinking, is vulnerable to conditioning. Maneuvering through these psycho-social-biological functions combined with the personal conditioning we absorb along the way creates our thinking ruts, or samskaras. Samskaras are entrenched ways of thinking and reacting that then become behavioral ruts too. These ruts become the most likely "go to,"

samskaras
and the six stations of the mind

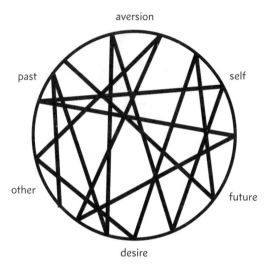

Figure 7.1

especially evident during robotic, alien-invader episodes. Often the ruts are so deep we don't even know we're in them, because we never experience ourselves as *not* in them. While our personal ruts will have their personal nuances, we are all subject to a universal obsession with specific mind patterns. For example, if you observe your own thought patterns for even a short amount of time, you will quite likely see yourself vacillating between past, future, self, other, aversion, and desire, what I call the "six stations of the mind." Embedded in our primitive brain, these vacillations occur at the level of the *manamayakosha,* along with our samskaras. Constantly ricocheting through the six stations may be our attempt to make sense of ourselves and our lives, yet it is also painfully distracting as we crowd out our ability to experience our deepest presence, contentment, ease, intuition, and the relief of the love, belonging, and joy that await us as we return to our center (remember the model of the koshas).

In addition to our personal samskaras, and the maze of our mind's six-station habits, we are also vulnerable to what yoga calls the *kleshas,* the five causes of suffering. These are powerful forces worth understanding, whether we're on the path to recovery from self-harming behaviors or addictions, or seeking to evolve psychologically or spiritually. Fortunately, yoga also teaches us that beneath the power of these strongly conditioned ways of being (including our disordered eating patterns) lies our intuition (vijnanamayakosha) and the strength to feel it, our creativity and the willingness to express it, and our psychological potential and the wisdom to live in relationship to it. Yoga's task is to help you get out of those brain ruts and awaken what's dormant. Your job in the journey of recovery is to stay aware of when you're moving from a place of conditioned mind or when you're moving from a place of wise mind.

At times recovery will feel terrifying as you are forced to challenge your conditioned mind (and consider new frontiers). At times, recovery feels like you might die (when old conditioning is dying). And at other times, it will feel like you're coming to life for the first time (when intuition and creativity are freed up)! The human organism is programmed with two competing imperatives: to survive and to thrive. From the perspective of your primitive brain, the six stations of the mind are primarily concerned with your survival: past aims to teach and protect you, future aims to lure you, self needs to be defended, others might be a threat. Aversions are to be avoided (they might be painful or cause death), and desires are to be pursued (they could extend life, or make it more pleasurable). As the primitive brain drives these reactions, it takes little to no conscious energy to engage in these processes. To decide to thrive requires energy, courage, rajas, and fervency. Based on the fact that you're reading this book, I'll hypothesize that living under the weight of survival structures that have covered over your thrive-ability isn't satisfying to you and that your urge to thrive is pushing your courage up to the surface to get your attention. It will either produce a phenomenal opening to your own potential, or, if untended or unheeded, it will produce a big mess.

How Much of Your Thinking Is Fresh?

How much of your thinking, then, is actually current with your life stage and your urge to be free from your outdated conditioning (which keeps you looping into your disordered eating patterns)? When we get triggered, we'll tend to react from the life stages we've been in; that is, we'll think the way we did when we were seven, or twelve, or sixteen. During our developmental years, we continually experience growth spurts, like the ones that got us to say "No!" or share our toys or recognize that Mommy and Daddy are separate from us. Although it takes about twenty-five years for the human brain to fully develop, life will still offer us opportunities for growth. Whether or not we're able to respond to them is an internal process, reflective of how our brains were formed in our early life. Fortunately, even though the brain completes its biologically programmed development by age twenty-five, we can keep growing through psycho-social-physical experiences that actively (and even passively) reshape us. Learning a foreign language, taking up the practices of yoga, developing creative pursuits, and learning new job tasks are all signs that the brain can still develop. However, the majority of our underlying conditioning is solidly in place by the time we're twenty-five. That means that unless we're conscious about it, the accumulation of the impressions, events, family and cultural messaging, and peer relationships that have shaped our brains before we're twenty-five have tremendous power. It's like the operating system on the hard drive of a computer. We can import and even update new software systems, but our hardwiring will still be our hardwiring.

Given this, you can understand why, even when you have compelling insight, a firm commitment, or even a medical urgency to create behavior change, it's still a tough thing to accomplish. Lasting behavior change will require fresh thinking and self-empathy. It doesn't require us to first dig up the sedimentary layers of the old thinking that created the behaviors. I understand this urge because it seems that if we could unravel the roots of our current painful behaviors, we would then be free of them. This is very tricky terrain to discuss because there are many schools of thought on this subject. Each offers a valid perspective. The perspective that I am bringing to this discussion is this: when we attempt to challenge the long-held beliefs of our conditioned mind, including our human vulnerability to the kleshas, we encounter conditioned mind's resistance to change. In this resistance we discover our history, our sedimentary layers, our six-station habits, our samskaras, and our humanity. How do we overcome this resistance and learn to shift to our wise mind's imperative for us to thrive and to grow into our potential, our 360-degree life? The yogic approach suggests that we can do this through understanding the kleshas and developing the tools to get free from their magnetic undertow.

KLESHAS: THE CAUSES OF HUMAN SUFFERING

The kleshas are the five most powerful and painful ways in which our minds become distorted and then cause us pain and suffering. These five causes of suffering are ignorance (*avidya*), ego (*asmita*), aversion (*dvesha*), desire (*raga*), and fear (*abhinivesha*). To work with the kleshas, we need to be able to successfully get in the GAP between the power of the kleshas to flood our brain space and the power of awareness to help us get grounded, employ attention, and return to presence. We must recruit our self-empathy and prevent the inner voice tone of shame. We must be willing to be uncomfortable for the sake of welcoming our spiritual imperative — to thrive — and we must be fervent enough that our biological imperative doesn't take over when we encounter the kleshas. Remember this: your biological imperative to survive and spiritual imperative to thrive cannot operate simultaneously. Your brain isn't set up for that. You must choose.

To prevent the five kleshas from charging up our biological drive, we practice the tools that develop the five kinds of joy. These are the joys that will continue to lay the pathway up the mountain out of our muddy ruts and switchbacks toward new horizons and capacity. These joys are of awe, belonging, tenderness, wholeness, and faith.

Avidya: *The Loss of Awe*

Avidya, the first klesha, is translated as ignorance, or the absence of wisdom. I interpret this as a state in which we have forgotten our basic nature, our deepest presence as love, consciousness, and oneness. In this condition, we misplace our deepest knowing and experience a loss of awe. In enters shame and the inner voice tone of shame. Essentially, the journeys of yoga and recovery are journeys out of this forgetfulness and back to deep remembrance, where we experience a profound sense of presence and love, self-empathy and acceptance, and an acknowledgment of the miracle that we exist.

> *Avidya is the state of forgetfulness, of not remembering, that causes a loss of awe.*
>
> *Awe is the state of wonder, humility, and appreciation about the miraculous in the ordinary, the preciousness of life.*

The loss of awe becomes a loss of self-respect. When we use disordered eating behaviors, we consistently disrespect the wisdom of our body, which was not meant to be a target for all the ways we try to contort it to the demands of our mind. Yet millions of people are at war with their body, appetite, size, cravings, and biological needs. When we start trying to control our appetite unnaturally, control the outcome of the size of our thighs, eat until we are ill or bloated, or force ourselves to burn all the calories we just ate, we're overriding the basic intelligence of our biology. Yoga wants you to live in harmony with your body. That means eating respectfully, exercising respectfully, and appreciating that your body has digestive, endocrine, and neurological programming that is designed to keep you functioning well. Loss of awe also means that we're more likely to forget our sense of deserving a vibrant, healthy, contented life. Yoga pulls us from forgetfulness to remember our innate worth and deservedness. And it pulls us into our lifeboat of self-empathy during shame floods.

The mental broadcasts that come through avidya will, by their very nature, cause suffering. The broadcasts will promote shame and body hatred, and thereby attempt to obstruct your intuition and self-respect. They will promote staying stuck in the sedimentary layers of old conditioning, and they will prevent you from risking new frontiers of thought and action. These broadcasts tend to be heavy, despairing, shaming, and reflect self-loathing. They question your worth and deny your beauty. The mental broadcasts of avidya will trigger your well-practiced FFFS response and threaten your ability to turn to your newly developing essential life skills for help.

❧ YOGA INQUIRY

Coming Back to Awe

Consistently come back to the state of awe that you exist. The practice:
- Acknowledge the precious news that you exist.
- Acknowledge that your body is breathing itself.
- Acknowledge that your heart is beating itself.
- Acknowledge that your eye lashes are growing themselves.
- Acknowledge that trees, birds, and weather patterns exist.
- Acknowledge that flowers come into bloom and apples ripen on trees.
- Acknowledge that something more powerful than your thoughts pushes crocuses up from the ground in late winter and creates the sky circles of birds in flight.
- This majesty is coursing through the blood in your veins, growing your hair, and blinking your eyes.
- This majesty has been in you all along, and is quietly awaiting your return.
- With a moment of quiet awe, give thanks.

~~ *Awe*

I've been listening to the "focus on awe" dharma talk by Sarahjoy during my commute to and from work. I am also practicing coping with anger, fear, and frustration emotions by softening, feeling connected to the source of these emotions (rooted in all humans), and creating space for my heart to fill. Between the "focus on the awe" practice and the softening, I now have useful ways to navigate through my interpersonal challenges—those that often spark the agitation that begs for comforting with food.

—*Diane, age 51*

Notice that the teachings suggest that you *consistently* reflect on the fact of your existence with an attitude of awe. You've already practiced the shame broadcast long enough. Therefore, you owe it to yourself to practice the awe broadcast for a dedicated period of time.

Awe cultivates a feeling of joy toward existence, including your own existence. This joy is not specifically personal toward any one thing. It is the joy we see also in hummingbirds and wild flowers.

Whatever you practice with repetition (yoga calls the chanting practice of repetition *japa*), your body-mind-psyche will be soaking it in. As I said, you've already soaked in the shame broadcast. That's made its impression in your body. As you practice the skill we are calling "coming back to awe," you may find that your physiology has a paradoxical response. On the one hand, you might feel a sense of relief, demonstrated by your heart rate or breathing rate slowing down. Yet, on the other hand, you may feel a sense of apprehension and disquiet, because you'll be challenging your old thought patterns. Remember when I said you didn't need to dig up your sedimentary layers, that in the process of making behavior changes you would encounter a resistance that tells you you're near to a discovery about your history? As you challenge old thought patterns, or samskaras, the disquiet you feel will reflect the source of those samskaras. Perhaps you'll feel that this repetition of continually coming back to awe isn't really applicable to you, or that it doesn't include you (maybe the bumblebees, but not you?), or that you could deserve it if you lost [a certain amount of] pounds first, or that it's silly and ineffective. However, I am still going to urge you to practice it. We become what we think. Therefore, attend to your thinking, use this practice to get in the GAP, and you will find yourself quietly evolving out of your old mental broadcasts.

 YOGA MOMENT

The Joy of Awe

To explore, through your body, the joy that arises toward life's preciousness, like the hummingbirds and wildflowers I mentioned before, we're going to use this yoga pose, the name of which, *anjaneyasana,* translates as "making an offering from the heart." It may be easier to embody this joy toward "the other," though I would like you to consider including yourself in your heart's offering as well.

ANJANEYASANA

Place your right foot forward and your left foot back in the basic lunge pose (p. 213). With your feet hip width apart from right to left, and with a stride long enough to keep your front shin vertical, touch your back knee down to the floor. If it is difficult to reach the floor with your fingers, use blocks. Then root

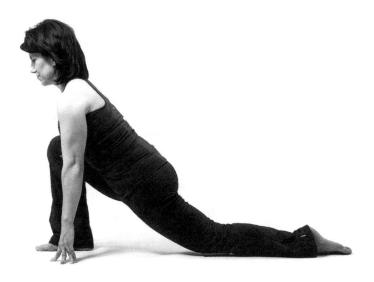

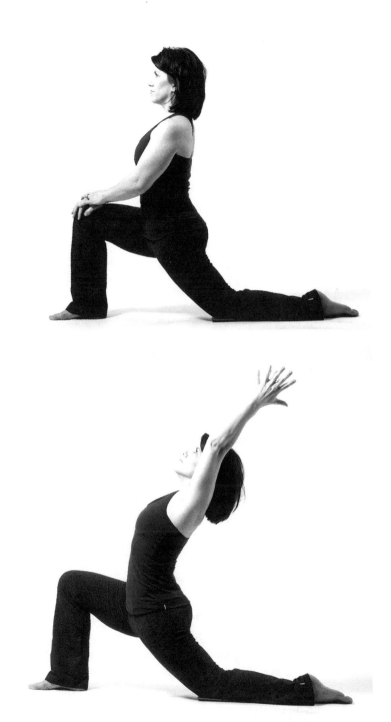

your tailbone so both your front foot and your back knee feel more grounded. Breathe evenly into your belly and bring to mind elements of life that remind you of what is precious, such as hummingbirds, the laughter of children, the dew on a rose petal. As you breathe, remind yourself that you are also an expression of awe in nature. When you are ready, inhale and shift your hands to your front knee.

Now, with an inhale, sweep your arms wide and up overhead placing your hands in a prayer position. Lift your heart and look up toward your palms. (You may find you're a bit off balance. This will get better with practice.) As you look up, aim to embody the quality of awe. Even if you have to pretend to feel this, you're waking up your body's memory of awe — which I am certain it experienced unabashedly at some moment in your life. (It may have gone underground until now, but the human heart's urge for the expression of delighted joy has not left you.)

Asmita: *The Loss of Belonging*

Asmita, or ego, means the making of a separate sense of self. I like to translate this klesha as a sense of separateness, isolation, or aloneness. Part of our human vulnerability reveals itself in our fear of being shunned, abandoned, betrayed, or rejected (we're programmed for it based on our early life dependence on others for our survival). Yet we're also capable of clever defense mechanisms. We may shut down caring about being included; we may become hardened by a protective shell intended to prevent feeling vulnerable to abandonment or rejection; we may puff up into arrogance; or we may develop our highly competent and indispensable side, to name a few common strategies.

Asmita is the painful experience of forgetting that we unconditionally belong.

Disordered eating patterns might start as a tool for self-soothing, as a way to regulate our emotions, or even as a way to keep ourselves company, yet one of their most painful side effects is the feeling of utter aloneness that can set in when we feel we are uniquely inept, crazy, or pathetic (just a few of the ways in which we talk to ourselves about this!). In isolation, shame has much more power. When we're vulnerable to internalizing shame, we're more likely to initiate survival skills that become defense mechanisms that then become addictions and compulsions. From the vantage point of the distorted lens of shame, what we're doing actually makes some sense. We've internalized shame into our "system," which is programmed for the biological imperative to survive. So we'll do what we have to in order to survive. To survive painful experiences, we'll reach for things that bring on the most immediate relief, even when those things are self-harming or go against the psycho-spiritual imperative of the human being: to realize itself, to evolve, to thrive, to remember that its basic nature is love itself.

Disordered eating patterns then heighten our sense of isolation. They carry too much shame, are too debilitating to permit clear thinking, require us to keep separating from the wisdom of our body and mind, and prevent our psycho-spiritual growth. Disordered eating patterns promote a sense of aloneness. Of course, as motivated as the human organism is to belong, people with addiction often can find a sense of belonging among other people with shared addictions. This doesn't tend to be the case with disordered eating patterns, though there are exceptions. We're more likely to see cigarette smokers, alcohol users, and gamblers building a sense of community around their substance or activity.

Without a doubt, the gift of regaining your sense of self-worth and returning to a genuine sense of deep belonging will be more satisfying than what addiction can do for you now.

YOGA INQUIRY

Returning to Belonging

A couple of things to understand about asmita, the "I" maker, or the ego: many of us were unable to develop a healthy sense of self out of the experiences of our early life. We may have poor differentiation skills, or difficulty knowing where we end and others begin. We may be prone to negating our own needs and tending to others. We may feel flooded by other people's emotions. And so we might hold tightly to the ego structure that we now have, even if it's surrounded by our fear, controlled by our body weight, or locked into thoughts about food and dieting. That distorted ego structure may be all we know.

The practice I'm going to suggest here is intended to widen your sense of belonging while also centering you in your own deserved self. Be aware that shame would tell you not to embark on this journey.

The practice we will call "returning to belonging" is a meditation practice of opening into wider circles of connection to others. It can be used as a daily seated meditation practice and is also portable and efficient. In other words, you can use it at any moment throughout the day.

- Clear your mind with three deep breaths. Give your attention to these breath cycles completely. Use the breaths to cross the threshold from thinking to presence.
- Now, bring to mind the countless seen and unseen others who are struggling with body-centered anxiety or self-hatred.
- Know that you are not alone.
- Extend wishes of well-being to these seen and unseen others.
- May they be free from suffering. May they gain knowledge, self-awareness, and self-empathy.
- Take another deep breath to clear your mind.
- Now, bring to mind all those seen and unseen others who are struggling with feeding themselves with self-respect.
- Know that you are not alone.
- Extend wishes of well-being to these seen and unseen others.
- May they be free from suffering. May they gain knowledge, self-awareness, and self-empathy.
- Now, bring to mind all those seen and unseen others who long for greater freedom from anxiety or depression.
- Know that you are not alone.
- Extend wishes of well-being to these seen and unseen others.
- May they be free from suffering. May they gain knowledge, self-awareness, and self-empathy.
- Now, bring to mind all those seen and unseen others, over the course of generations and across spiritual traditions, who are practicing to wake up out of suffering. Bring to mind all those seen and unseen others who will sit in meditation, light a candle, contemplate their mental patterns, breathe and move their bodies prayerfully, chant, and so on.
- Know that you are not alone.
- Extend wishes of well-being to these seen and unseen others.
- May they be free from suffering. May they gain knowledge, self-awareness, and self-empathy.
- Now, bring yourself to mind. May you be free from suffering. May you gain knowledge, self-awareness, and self-empathy.

Returning to belonging invites us to feel a quiet joy about our place in the family of life. The joy of belonging has qualities of quietude, simplicity, and restfulness, like mountain streams carrying the glacial runoff to the ocean.

YOGA MOMENT

The Joy of Belonging

Inherently, belonging invites us to release the striving we demand of ourselves to prove or demonstrate our worth, or to keep ourselves painfully walled in to our personal shame-dungeon. In yoga poses, we use a quality of relaxed effort. There should be nothing aggressive about these efforts, even when a pose demands that you participate in a strong or thoughtful manner (as when lifting away from gravity, for example, in cobra pose, below).

COBRA AND CHILD'S POSE

Cobra is a heart-opening pose that also strengthen the upper back posture muscles. Child's pose is a pose of inwardness and refuge.

Lie on your stomach and place your hands beneath your shoulders. Root your tailbone down toward the floor and engage your leg muscles. Momentarily rest your head on the floor in a gesture of humility. Inhale into your belly and as you exhale press yourself up to cobra pose. While breathing smoothly, extend your heart forward, without jutting your chin out. Gaze toward the floor a few inches ahead of your pose. As you inhale, feel your breath connecting you to the ground beneath you; also feel it encouraging your heart to shine forward. With your exhale, release any sense of straining; acknowledge that you belong and that your efforts are in the spirit of remembering that. Spend several moments breathing in the feeling of your sense of quietude and belonging.

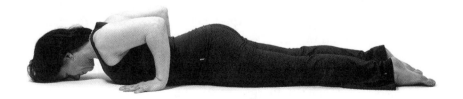

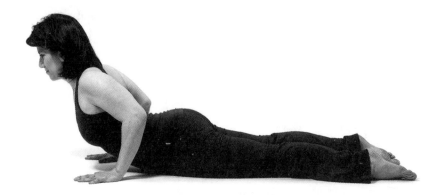

With an inhale, press yourself up and back to child's pose. Bring your hips toward your heels. Keep your arms outstretched and feel the energy of your body easing into the floor and the energy of your heart flowing downstream from your upper back, through your arms and hands, into the floor and beyond, the way a mountain stream carries itself gracefully, humbly, downward.

Dvesha: *The Loss of Tenderness*

Dvesha means aversion or hatred. It can range from aversion to the weather or to people's personality quirks; to the sense of loathing about our thighs, freckles, cellulite, or hair texture; to deep-seated revulsion toward the fact that we exist. In disordered eating and addiction, we've tried to use self-hatred to condemn, motivate, control, and punish. We've learned to use hatred to harm ourselves, to deepen the shame.

In order to actively hate something about ourselves, we would already have lost our ability to feel tenderness toward ourselves. Shame provokes self-hatred. We know that feeling already. Shame can also take the shape of hatred toward, or revulsion about, others. Many people with body image issues, for example, have an experience of revulsion toward other people's fat as well as their own (real or perceived). Surprisingly, shame can also show up as hatred toward people we perceive as beautiful according to our cultural standards. We learn to hate someone else's perfect hair, or we'll hate them for having cellulite-free legs or blemish-free skin. Dvesha promotes opportunities to hate ourselves in the form of self-condemnation for our perceived flaws or envy for what we deem to be other people's perfections.

Dvesha is the state of self-hatred that blocks our self-tenderness.

What if, toward all hatred and all derivations of hatred, we were to practice tenderness toward ourselves and others instead?

Here's something that may be easy for you to relate to, given your relationship to food or body image, but it can seem baffling to those who have not experienced it. When we are in a shame storm of self-condemnation, let's say toward the shape of our thighs or the size of our belly, we can experience palpable annoyance, anger, and hatred toward the specific body part or toward ourselves as a whole. And then, in response to that anger and hatred, we'll actively do something that actually makes it all worse. Bingeing on ice cream or angrily eating corn chips in response to how we look in the mirror or what we weigh on the scale doesn't make any rational sense. Yet it makes sense at the level of where we're actually in pain.

When we lose our sense of awe and belonging, we lose our sense of worth and deservedness. This is the pain that is deeper than our flawed thighs. But hating our flawed thighs feels more manageable than hating something we can't name or control: shame, the family systems that perpetuate shame, and a culture that uses shame to motivate, control, and reinforce emptiness.

We will also hate our thighs because, if they are "imperfect," we know, deep down, that they are the reason that we deserve punishment. We are trying to blot out or overcome the thing that makes us feel shame. Yet, rather than direct our rage at the source of our pain (shame), we direct it at something that we feel we can do something about: our body, body parts, appetite, and so on.

Remember when I said that until we're provoked by a growth spurt we'll use the thinking we've been using, even if it resembles our thinking when we were seven, twelve, or sixteen? Well, this experience of body-centered self-hatred is your provocative growth spurt. If you still think that hating your thighs, or eating out of anger at the scale, or bingeing in response to how tight your jeans are makes some sense, then you are invited to radically alter how you think about your body, your anger, and your self-hatred.

You don't need to go forward being so vulnerable to the chronically disappointing self-assessments that shame provides. You deserve to live in awe about the fact that you exist. And you deserve to reconnect to your sense of belonging. Your self-hatred broadcast needs to be drowned out by your self-tenderness broadcast!

⤳ YOGA INQUIRY

Awakening Self-Tenderness

For your recovery from self-harm, it is absolutely essential that you cultivate an attitude of what we will call "awakening self-tenderness." This is the tenderness you would naturally extend to yourself if shame weren't in the way. This tenderness will not cause you to become a slothful couch potato, nor will it make you weak. This tenderness is the kind of tenderness you would extend toward a wounded animal, an elderly person making an effort to rise from a chair and judging themselves for their difficulty, or a small child with an illness who feels there is something wrong with him for being sick. (*Notice whether you're feeling resistance right now. If so, take three deep breaths, put aside that thought broadcast, and keep reading.*) To extend tenderness toward that which is vulnerable, wounded, fragile, or hurting initiates healing. Sadly, you learned to extend shame toward your vulnerability or frustration toward your fragility. You probably thought this was a useful way to overcome vulnerability, protect yourself from harm (from others), or prevent yourself from causing further shame to yourself.

The practice of awakening self-tenderness is initially directed toward yourself and to the many ways in which hatred has overwhelmed your self-tenderness. It will ripple out to others. You will find your compassion growing.

- Toward the part of my thighs that I hate: I offer myself tenderness for the pain that hating my thighs causes. May I be free from this kind of pain.
- Toward the part of my skin that I hate: I offer myself tenderness for the pain that hating my skin causes. May I be free from this kind of pain.
- Toward the size of my belly: I offer myself tenderness for the pain that hating my belly causes. May I be free from this kind of pain.
- Toward my cellulite, stretch marks, skin blemishes, or scars: I offer myself tenderness for the pain that hating my cellulite, stretch marks, skin blemishes, or scars causes. May I be free from this kind of pain.
- Toward the part of me that gets frustrated: I offer myself tenderness for the pain that hating my frustration causes. May I be free from this kind of pain.
- Toward the part of me that flares up in anger toward myself: I offer myself

tenderness for the pain that hating my anger causes. May I be free from this kind of pain.

- Toward the part of me that I incessantly evaluate as failing: I offer myself tenderness for the pain that hating my self-evaluations causes. May I be free from this kind of pain.
- Toward the part of me that gets overwhelmed: I offer myself tenderness for the ways in which I get overwhelmed. May I be free from this kind of pain.
- Toward the part of me that has been ruled by shame: I offer myself tenderness for the pain that shame causes. May I be free from this kind of pain.

Tenderness is one of the capacities of the human heart that opens us to healing. It can be stirred by our own pain or by exposure to the pain of another, to which we may feel how precious, how fleeting, how tender life is. Being able to experience tenderness strengthens our heart's ability to feel. The joy of tenderness allows us to respond with heart when we encounter pain. It also lets us feel the pain of being tenderly and completely accepted. It is gentle and respects how fragile things may shy away from too-forceful efforts toward joy. It is like sunrises in the winter.

YOGA MOMENT

The Joy of Tenderness

To experience the joy of tenderness in your body, it helps to practice directing your energy both inwardly and outwardly. Alternating between turning inward toward those parts of you that have been in pain and turning outward toward your participation in life (and toward life's acceptance of you) awakens your ability to be tender with yourself while also releasing the weight of self-hatred, dvesha.

CAT AND COW POSE

Place yourself on all fours. For the cat pose, press down through both arms and round your spine toward the ceiling, like a Halloween cat. Bring your head down between your upper arms and direct your attention inwardly. Breathe slowly into the back hemisphere of your body several times, allowing the back of the waist and heart to release tension. Simultaneously, imagine yourself scooping out the belly with each exhale, releasing the residue of self-hatred that blocks you from breathing well. Do this five or six times.

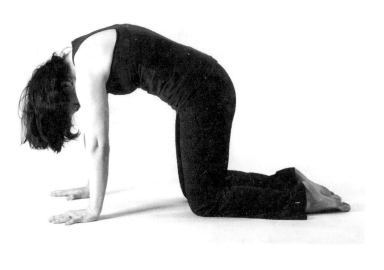

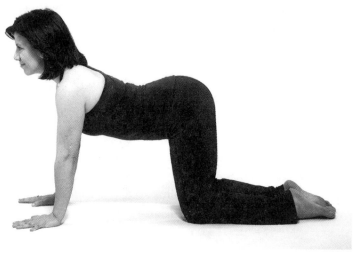

Now, inhale and bring your spine to cow pose by arching your back and extending your heart forward. This is called cow pose because the spine reflects the shape of the arched back of the cow. As you breathe deeply into your belly, extend your attention outward toward your participation in life. Even if the upper back or the heart ache in doing this, consider it a healing ache, like the pain of frostbite when it is thawing. As you continue to breathe,

❧ Self-Tenderness, not Self-Hatred

I'm responding to this binge with more self-compassion and efforts at awareness. The binge was definitely triggered by exhaustion and delayed eating from a busy day. I wasn't honoring my vitality and I let my personal buoyancy get pretty deflated. Sometimes I feel like being gentle with myself is the same as telling myself it's okay and then feeling like I will never break this cycle. I know the triggers, I know how awful the next day feels, and yet these days reoccur. I'm trying to regroup by adjusting parts of my schedule to lessen the triggers and set myself up for better things—for feeling more like me. But truthfully, I'm forever surprised by where she went in looking at myself caught in this disordered eating. I feel like no one outside of our group understands the mind trap involved here. For example: I want to exercise to feel better, but my body feels awful so it's hard to exercise. I want to eat better, but when bingeing there's just a pervasive "I don't care, just finish it so it's gone" mentality, so that it can feel like small victories are very far away. Today it is a new day. I got more sleep. And I am trying to go from here with continued compassion and self-tenderness. I already know self-hatred doesn't work.

—Amanda, age 27

soften the upper back a bit more, and extend your heart forward with the joy of tenderness (remember, do not be aggressive; aggression makes shy things back away).

Now slowly alternate between the two poses, inhaling for cat pose and exhaling for cow pose.

Raga: *The Loss of Wholeness*

Raga, or the klesha of desire, is passionate grasping for something. It can range from desire for a lemonade, a new car, or the perfect life, or thinness, control, or perfection. Yet desire also runs away with us—for instance, on occasions when a quart of ice cream is demolished in a few minutes' time.

When the human mind is in a state of desire, it quite literally feels that what it seeks will complete it or bring it back to satisfaction. Feelings of emptiness provoke desire. Feelings of incompleteness provoke grasping. Feelings of brokenness provoke urgency. Whether this is urgency for attaining a specific appearance or eating a restricted number of calories, or an unmitigated binge on bread and pasta, we're attempting to satisfy a particular restlessness that arises for all human organisms when they have lost their wholeness.

> *Raga is the undercurrent of incessant restlessness as we try to find our way back to wholeness.*

Of course, from the time we are born, we're always developing and growing. Yet the concept of wholeness that I'm pointing to here doesn't imply completeness, in the sense of finishing. To those of you with perfectionistic streaks, I'm sure you've noticed that you don't actually get to arrive at a perfectly controlled body moment and then keep it that way! The human organism is always unfolding and evolving, and it is incapable of permanently fixed biological states. Yet, I understand the urge to craft something solid to hold on to. Paradoxically, the spiritual teachings that I have discovered over the past twenty-five years all suggest this truth: there is no solid thing to hold on to. Addiction and disordered eating strategies are crafted to give us this sense of something to hold on to amid an otherwise vast and unknowable ocean.

To those of you who use compulsive eating to fill an unidentifiable, insatiable void, I'm sure you've also noticed that the satiation never lasts. The void doesn't actually ever say, "Thank you. That will do it. Enough." It can be profoundly frustrating to realize this — or it can be liberating. When we can bring tenderness to the part of us that has made up these strategies, we will be able to stop damning ourselves long enough to feel another underlying reality, a paradoxically and equally true reality:

You have always been whole. You were born into wholeness. And nothing can cause that to be diminished or broken. The only thing between you and this knowing is your thinking.

I didn't experience this sense of wholeness until I took up the practices of yoga. Then, fortunately, it took a while before I had experiences of this kind of mystical, vibrating wholeness. I say "fortunately" because otherwise I would have scared myself away from yoga! However, when I did experience it, I was ready. It was remarkably soothing and quieted a part of my mind that had become painful. Of course, the experience of wholeness didn't last; it came and went. It came on triggered by my yoga practice, and then left again, triggered by my thinking, anxiety, and fear.

I think it's worthwhile to detour here to spend a moment on the differences among emptiness, fullness, and wholeness, specifically related to food addiction and disordered eating patterns.

I understand the longing for the feeling of emptiness that comes from food restriction rituals and from purging. Yoga also has practices related to diet, including fasting. The feelings of lightness, cleanness, and clearheadedness, and the very real sensations of emptiness, can induce a sense of quiet spiritual connectedness. Yet the emptiness won by food restriction or purging is very different from the physiological clarity of a clean yogic diet or short periods of supervised fasting. The emptiness associated with anorexia isn't usually associated with a deeply relaxed nervous system but rather with feelings of rigidity, control, or anxiety. In fact, at a certain body weight, your physiology will have to undergo biochemical changes related to starvation and preservation. These side effects are very different from the benefits of a yogic diet, because they arise from a violent act on the part of the body. Although the body's ability to purge toxic food on its own, voluntarily, is indeed a cleansing of sorts, it is also, by nature, the body's attempt to violently, immediately expel something toxic. When we induce vomiting, as in bulimic patterns, we're imposing an unnatural violence on the body. Often tied to the rush of the binge part of the cycle, the emptiness that follows this is more closely related to feeling wrung out, numbed, or relieved of the urgency that preceded the binge-purge. Yet your brain chemistry will go out of balance, and your body will experience a level of malnourishment with this cyclical and disruptive behavior.

It would be remiss of me not to address this aspect of our conversation, because I know that many of us who have used disordered eating strategies may be seeking that feeling of emptiness and trying to avoid the uncomfortable feelings of fullness. The feeling of fullness for some of us is scary; for others among us it is the only time that we feel a sense of relief from our underlying anxieties, mental broadcasts, or shame. Compulsive overeating, eating past the point of fullness, and bingeing dismiss the innate intelligence of the body. While some of us may be looking to fill a void, overcome painful feelings of emptiness, or buffer ourselves from the vulnerabilities of life, these food-based strategies don't lead to feelings of wholeness. Even if the void gets filled for a few hours, it will gnaw at us again. Even if we overcome the psychological pain of our isolation or emptiness, loss of awe, and loss of belonging, the food we ingest will not fix it or make it better, ever.

Wholeness, on the other hand, is a feeling of nothing missing, nothing broken, nothing gnawing at the mind, body, or heart. The experience of wholeness is closely related to the physiological state of deep relaxation, centering, presence, or ease. It includes feelings of safety and faith in who we are and how we are growing. At the same time, it isn't dependent on having all the right or perfect circumstances, such as getting good grades, a raise at our job, or the recognition of five thousand Facebook fans. This wholeness underlies all of that. It is related to the dignity a person can feel in spite of mistreatment or injustice. (It doesn't preclude having appropriately angry responses.) It is also related to the sense of intactness a person feels in her being even if she breaks her arm, loses a limb, or becomes paralyzed. Nothing can impact this felt wholeness.

These distinctions among emptiness, fullness, and wholeness are fundamental to your recovery. Once we've lost our sense of awe (avidya), our sense of belonging (asmita), and our sense of tenderness (dvesha), we're profoundly vulnerable. This lost sense of wholeness produces desire: the grasping and urgency of the hungry ghosts that pull us to and fro, creating a chronically anxious state. Paradoxically, you will fight against this constructed arrangement, even sabotaging your own (shame-based) food plans to do so, because the wholeness that you are and that longs to express itself through you does not want you to be punished by that which goes against the ingrained intelligence of your human body and its right to be here.

✒ YOGA MOMENT

Reconnecting to Wholeness

As with all of the meditations in this chapter, these practices are intended to teach you the skill of getting in the GAP, getting grounded, wielding attention, and returning to presence. Each of them momentarily GAPs your mind, by giving it a specific focus, quieting its mental broadcast, or shaking it out of its self-recrimination spell. Although this is an active meditation, it is still portable. The second breathing practice may feel awkward to do in public, but finding a discreet opportunity when you need it is a way of rallying for your recovery!

Progressive Muscle Relaxation with Breath Retention

This involves three steps:
1. Inhale deeply and hold the breath.
2. Squeeze every possible muscle in your body.
3. Exhale slowly and deliberately.

Inhale deeply and hold the breath:

Take a very deep breath in through your nose, slowly, deeply, fully. Hold the breath in for a short count. During this time, consciously expand your breath out against the skin of your body and fill yourself up completely. If you were a balloon, you will be as expanded as possible from the inside. As you do this, also imagine pressing all of the tension out of your body and mind, sending thoughts and feelings out for a temporary vacation.

Squeeze every possible muscle in your body:

While holding the breath in, squeeze every muscle tight, including your eyes, your face, and even your hands (which you can make into fists). This will have the effect of squeezing the balloon-like state you have put your inner body into. It is like a giant hug from your skin and muscles against your breath and bones. Squeeze like you are squeezing a sponge to press all the excess water out. Wring out your muscles and your mind fully.

Exhale slowly and deliberately:

After holding the breath-squeeze for up to ten seconds, exhale slowly, over the course of ten seconds. It might help to time this the first few times you try it. While exhaling, picture yourself releasing all of the tension and holding of your mind and body, the way a baby kitten goes limp when it's mother picks it up from the back of the neck. At the end of the exhale, allow for the natural pause and listen quietly for the stillness.

Repeat this three times. At the end of three rounds you will have reduced the physiological tightness of your mind and body. You will also have explored states of fullness, tightness, emptiness, and ease. In the resolution of the tension, you will be able to glimpse your innate, unbreakable wholeness. That wholeness has been there all along; it is your birthright. It exists simply because you exist. You didn't have to earn it, but you do have to remember it.

Alternate Nostril Breathing

Using your right thumb and ring finger, you will alternately inhale and exhale through the left and right nostrils. The pattern is:

inhale left   exhale right
inhale right   exhale left

This is considered one round of alternate nostril breathing. This breath cycle brings together the right and left hemispheres of the brain, cleanses the nervous system, slows down your breathing, and calms the mind.

Sit up straight.

Bring your right hand up to your nose, with the index and middle fingers tucked in. Using your right thumb, close the right nostril and *inhale left*. Then using your right ring finger, close your left nostril and *exhale right*. Now, *inhale right*. Then, using your right thumb, close your right nostril and *exhale left*.

Repeat this for four rounds (eight breaths).

Then sit quietly and explore the sense of wholeness and your place in the larger pulse of nature.

Radiance is an energetic force that moves outward (as in radiating), ignited by a central force. It can also be the result of unblocking or removing an obstacle that has suppressed a radiant force. The joy of wholeness is nonurgent, nonstriving. It is the wholeness that shines through when we unblock the tensions of our mind or body. It is the quality of shine we see when the sun makes it through the canopy to the leaves on the forest trees. It is also the way the leaves accept this shine, without fanfare or urgency.

 ## YOGA MOMENT

The Joy of Wholeness

The joy of wholeness does not rely on us feeling our absolute best. It does, however, correlate with us being more deeply rested and centered. Though this joy has a quality of shine, it is not driven by adrenaline. It is more of an inner glow.

Reclined Supported Backbend

For this exercise you will need a bolster and a folded blanket. Lie back on the bolster, allowing it to support your lumbar curve, chest, and head. (To

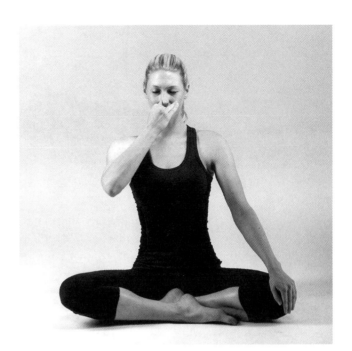

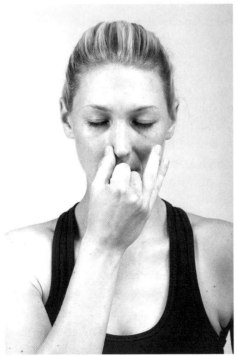
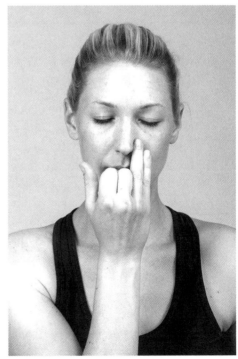

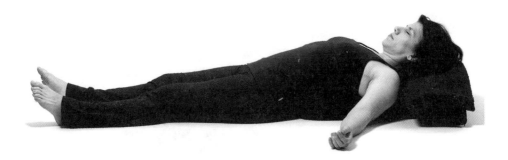

substitute for a bolster, you may use a couple of folded blankets, neatly arranged.) Then set up the blanket under your head to prop it up so that you have the sense that you are gazing inwardly toward your heart. (In this position, your forehead will not tip backward.) Invite your legs to relax.

Allow yourself to rest in this position for a minimum of six minutes. Ten to twelve minutes will make a more profound impact on your nervous system and, thus, your inner wholeness.

Abhinivesa: *The Loss of Faith*

Abhinivesa, or fear, is fear of death. We all know we will someday die, and we know that someday all the people and things that we care about will die, too. Losing our sense of awe, belonging, tenderness, and wholeness already represents several important deaths. The fear of death is programmed into the human organism. Even if you were a high-level Zen meditation student, you would still experience a physiological rush if your airplane were in terrible weather with a mechanical malfunction.

On the spiritual journey, as with other areas of human development and adventure, we will experience the death of old ways of being, previous protective mechanisms, negative aspects of our self-image, self-imposed limitations, and the conditioning that once defined us. These deaths lead to feelings of liberation. For example, if you were convinced by others that you could not sing (and perhaps that you *should* not sing!), and you decided to take singing lessons, or even start robustly singing spontaneously, you would set in motion an opportunity to die to an old way of being, an old message, an old part of your self-image. The courage to do this represents the part of you that has not lost hope. That part is willing to be frightened in order to take advantage of the opportunity to grow. When fear causes us to lose motivation, suppress our hopes, and pretend that nothing matters, it shrinks our 360-degree life and furthers the belief that we should be afraid.

> *Abhinivesa is the fear of dying to old ways of being.*
> *It is the loss of faith that fear is an opportunity to grow.*

To overcome the ways in which we've suppressed ourselves, given in to conditioning, and been led by our fear away from opportunity or intimacy will require faith in the process. As we take the steps to grow, we will be outgrowing our shell, like the baby chick. Yet to us it will feel like dying. We may actually feel terrified and even have sweaty palms. (This is where the tool of checking in with your physiology through dashboarding becomes important.) Under the guidance of a skilled therapist, this temporary death becomes a birth into new awareness, new ways of being, and new capacity to follow through on our insights.

We will need faith to prevent us from getting sidetracked and to remind us of three things:

1. Something in you wants to make this journey. (Remember, the fight or struggle you're having with yourself demonstrates that.)
2. Your physiology is intelligently programmed and sending you signals to use for your journey. (Learning to tune in to your physiology will help you trust yourself. Remember that fear and excitement produce very similar physiological states.)
3. There is a magnetic pull to the yoga broadcast, and it is ultimately stronger than the magnetic pull of the shame broadcast. (It is stronger because it is true. Shame has never told you the truth.)

As you rebuild your faith in fear as an opportunity to grow, keep in mind that it will feel counterintuitive. Fear is meant to trigger our fight-flight-freeze-submit response for personal preservation. One of your most used self-preservation strategies has been your disordered eating patterns. We both know that strategy is not working and it's not producing the intended outcome. Our lives actually get smaller, harder, more vulnerable, and more exhausting under the influence of addiction. So you'll have to reorient to the notion that when you feel fear, you're being given a chance to grow. Your breath, your mindfulness, and your mental broadcast station will be major contributors to whether or not you choose fear as a way to grow or whether you let fear tell you to be more frightened.

Another critical aspect of faith is your faith in yourself. We looked at this in depth in chapter 5, but to repeat briefly, your faith in yourself has been damaged by your disordered eating patterns. Now, looking through the new lens offered in this book, you can rework your understanding of this "failure." In the past, you made efforts out of the shame broadcast. Most likely the strategies you came up with were not in harmony with your body's intelligence. FFFS patterns and self-preservation samskaras are primal and powerful grooves in the mind. Remember that every time you rebel against yourself represents an important inner conflict: between the part of you that *must* grow, that is living out its imperative to move toward your 360-degree life, and the part of you that has been using shame to create minimizing life strategies and avert what it perceives as "danger."

During periods of recovery, when your symptoms increase, rather than damn yourself as having another failure, consider this:

1. Some part of you feels like it is in danger.
2. If it is your fundamental well-being, your self-preservation or survival strategies will kick in.
3. If you don't have new and well-established tools to use, you'll go back to what has worked.
4. Once you start doing this, the part of you that wants recovery, the recovery of your *whole* life, will push into the conflict and make you feel restless. This is a healthy agitation; it's flagging your attention that something is out of balance.
5. In the rise or return of symptoms, you can bet that your fear mechanism just got set off. It's either an external fear, such as conflict in your social environment telling your animal instinct that you aren't safe, or an internal fear, such as the fear of moving forward in your recovery and having to use your new getting-comfortable-feeling-uncomfortable skills to face painful emotions.

In all of this, it is utterly critical that you learn how to invoke faith over fear. Your faith in yourself is understandably weak right now. Faith in that fear is also understandably counterintuitive. However, I'll bet you've tried some other unusual things to get yourself out of pain.

YOGA INQUIRY

Invoking Faith

Yoga teaches us that there are three kinds of faith that we can apply here:
- *astikya*: faith in the science and teachings of yoga, as taught by our "ancestor yogis"
- *mati*: faith in ourselves when yoga is applied to our life; will
- *shradda*: faith in the underlying intelligence of life

Let's translate that into recovery terms:
- faith in the process of recovery, as passed down by those who have made it out
- faith in yourself, your sense of belonging and worth, your deservedness for recovery, and your capacity to do it
- faith in an underlying intelligence in life
Here are some ways you can explore each one.

Faith in the Process of Recovery

- Read books and articles about people's successful recoveries.
- Attend meetings or group therapy, or develop friendships with people who are recovered or recovering.
- Read about the science of the brain and its capacity to change.
- Find a doctor, naturopath, or functional medicine nutritionist to help you understand the relationship between food and your brain.

Faith in Yourself

- Create your personal dashboard. Review the dashboarding exercise on page 197. Make a personal, visible representation of your dashboard, or download the Hunger, Hope, and Healing app to your phone or iPad (see Resources). Look at your dashboard often in order to embed your awareness of it in your mind.
- Make a personal list of the practices in this book (see "Practices and Short Sequences" on p. 283) to which you can commit.
- Reflect on the commitments you are able to keep. Do *not* focus on any "lack" or "less than." (You've already tried that method to motivate yourself.)

- Knowing that these practices will be able to overtake your old habits, keep moving toward your commitment with regular appreciation of your efforts.

On a seesaw, for every ounce moved from one end to the other, there is an incremental shift. While we can't see it initially, we know that, mathematically, it will happen. It is the same process with taking on the tools of your recovery.

Faith in an Underlying Intelligence in Life

- Spend time quietly in nature.
- Witness the sunrise, the sunset, or birds in flight. Feel the timelessness of these rhythms in life.
- Before eating, consciously return to a perspective of awe and appreciation that food grows itself. (Give praise to the broccoli! Give thanks for the orange groves!)
- Read about the power of the human spirit, especially the power that endures through suffering, injustice, or pain. Recall how many generations of human life have endured throughout history.

Recalling our collective, interdependent experience of life can pull us out of isolation and the primitive mind's imperative to scan through the six stations looking for fear. To remember our collective life is to become both less isolated and more trusting in life's larger unfolding. We experience the joy of faith in the larger collective of life, in nature and in humans. It is the joy infused in the interdependent web of life. It is fruit ripening, bees pollinating, humans journeying. It is life sustaining itself, moment to moment, over eons. When we feel this quality of joy, we recognize that life sustains and nourishes us; and that we are a part of the greater collective of life.

ᴖ YOGA INQUIRY

The Joy of Faith

To explore this joy as an innate experience of your humanity, I invite you to go outdoors, to walk among the trees, or experience the rain on your skin or the wind against your face, all entirely without agenda. Or immerse yourself in the marketplace of other people, without agenda. As an introvert, I shy away from crowded places. Yet when I walk with the intention to feel my collective humanity, I can walk among a community fair, a farmer's market, or the esplanade downtown in Portland and my introvert bubble is able to experience community without being flooded. If being amid other humans in that way isn't conducive at first, begin with nature. We can be quite still inside, as we step outside without an agenda, whether we are walking among our human family or among the trees. In that stillness, the maze of the mind settles down, the six stations and the kleshas fade, and what comes forward is the joy of faith in the larger collective.

Part Four

FORGIVENESS
and FREEDOM
(STAGE THREE)

8

FORGIVENESS
and FREEDOM

HERE WE ENTER THE THIRD STAGE OF RECOV-
ery, based on kriya yoga: surrender. This stage of recovery
is built on the strengths of fervency and the capacities of self-empathy, leading
us to surrender the pain we've been in as well as our outdated, painful behaviors. For the purpose of recovery, I teach this as forgiveness and freedom.

FORGIVENESS

Let's start a very important application of forgiveness: self-forgiveness. As with
all the other tools and skills in this book, self-forgiveness becomes a support
beyond getting out of cycles of disordered eating and adds tremendously to
the value and depth of life. Very few of us know how to practice self-forgiveness. Self-forgiveness repairs your self-respect, prevents self-shame, deepens
your self-empathy, and opens you to learn from whatever error, slip, or stumble you've made.

Responding to a "Slip" with Self-Forgiveness

- Self-forgiveness recognizes that your mind and your current life skills are
  the result and reflection of all previous life events and conditioning. With
  this recognition, you surrender the self-blame that shame wants to use to
  further reinforce your "badness."
- Self-forgiveness sees your earnestness in every attempt to recover, to self-
  soothe, to grow, and to learn, even when you've made less than skillful choices.

- Self-forgiveness means you don't hold yourself hostage to "the things you've done." You surrender the concept that you are perpetually trying to make up for the "bad" you've done or been.
- Self-forgiveness creates a learnable brain state, not a frightened one (fright is a state from which we can't actively learn).
- Self-forgiveness sees you as constantly on the path toward wholeness, even when you experience a "slip" or "setback."
- At its deepest, self-forgiveness is a statement to ourselves that we will not self-abandon. We will not be the source of shunning or banishment of ourselves. Under any circumstances.

Self-forgiveness is not lazy nor self-indulgent. It is not a means to deception or manipulation. Those are symptoms of shame-thinking. Remember that self-recrimination stirs survival mechanisms, fight-flight-freeze-submit functions, and self-preservation strategies. It creates the physiology of defending against growth. Self-forgiveness produces an inner environment of moving from love, not shame. In this brain and body state, we have room for learning something new, remembering recently acquired skills or insights, developing the skill of foresight, avoiding painful setbacks, and deepening our sense of connection to and respect for ourselves. Because of the impact that self-forgiveness has physiologically, it enables us to (1) recognize what we've done or are about to do (the error or stumble), (2) see it in a larger context (a symptom of an imbalance, for example), (3) make use of hindsight, present sight, and foresight, (4) resist urges for harmful self-talk, and (5) follow learning curves toward greater capacity and commitment. In these ways self-forgiveness builds the fortitude we need for the journey of recovery, the recovery of our 360-degree life.

1. *Recognize what we've done or are about to do:* They say hindsight is 20/20. That means we are often able to see more clearly after an experience than before or during it. Yet the skills you are learning in recovery also produce your ability for present sight and foresight. Whether you see yourself using unskillful choices in hindsight, see yourself moving toward self-harming behavior as it's happening, or recognize the physiological and psychological vulnerabilities that could lead you to act unwisely, each of these involves seeing yourself. Look through the lens of love, not shame. Self-forgiveness for a stumble picks you up faster than shame will. Self-forgiveness in the moment you're opening the binge food helps you put it down. And self-forgiveness for letting

your physiological or psychological well-being become vulnerable prevents you from self-abandoning and restores your safe and secure connection with yourself.

2. *See it in a larger context:* Living into your recovery, daily, weekly, on an ongoing basis, you will come to see your thoughts and actions in a larger context. It's far less probable that you can justify punishing yourself with shame when you see your behavior in the larger context of your life. The larger context might include the social milieu you're in, your schedule or routine, your responsibilities or the demands on you, your particular vulnerabilities or triggers, and how your physiology is responding to all of those influences. You are not going to be perfectly balanced in your physiology all the time. However, you can consistently respond to your slips with self-nurturance, self-respect, self-empathy, and self-forgiveness to help bring you back to making healthy choices for rest, renewal, nourishment, and physiological balance.

3. *Make use of hindsight, present sight, and foresight:* Loving hindsight helps you realize a different choice you could have made. For example, give the symphony tickets away and go home early for good rest. Or say "no thank you" to a summer barbeque and potluck that might put you in a too-vulnerable situation. Or eat a healthy meal before going to the barbeque so you'll be less likely to be too hungry to think well about possible trigger foods. Present sight (that is, seeing yourself in the present moment) helps restore clarity, as when you see yourself making the purchase of unhealthy foods and realize you're on your trajectory. You can make a course correction right in that moment. Foresight helps you recognize that when your physiology or psychology is out of balance you're much more vulnerable to old habits, including thinking habits. Foresight can be self-correcting, as you plan to go for a walk in the park or take a hot bath to restore yourself.

4. *Resist urges for harmful self-talk:* Through recovery, you've explored the inner voice of shame and its intent to promote self-harm. Knowing the damage this inner voice can do, you resist harmful self-talk by replacing it with self-empathy, with kindness, and with recruiting "gray area" thinking (not shame and addiction's black-and-white, good-and-bad strategies). Thinking in the gray area is one of the tools of yogic surrender, placing you on the path toward freedom. The gray area is fundamental to the teachings of what we will call "first do less harm, then do more good."

5. *Follow learning curves toward greater capacity and commitment:* Moving through 1, 2, 3, and 4, you place yourself in a learning curve, the opposite of

a hairpin turn back toward shame and powerlessness. A conscious learning curve pulls you along the trajectory toward increased capacity to have leadership over your recovery and to deepen your commitment to your 360-degree life. These learning curves act like the fun-to-drive-through curves on an open road wherein we pick up speed as we exit the curve and experience the feeling of ease and direction, the movement toward another aspect of the experience of yogic surrender: freedom.

A Self-Forgiveness and Freedom Essential: "First Do Less Harm, Then Do More Good"

When faced with possible slips, flushes, or upheavals in your recovery, the approach we will call "first do less harm, then do more good" is a step-by-step process to preserve your two toeholds, revive your courage, and reinforce self-forgiveness. With all potential flushes or upheavals, there will be an accompanying thought-storm that tries to move us to black-and-white thinking. When we undertake to "first do less harm, then do more good," we use self-forgiveness to demote black-and-white thinking, recognizing that an absolute approach such as good-bad thinking can never be successful. It cannot be successful because (1) it is adversarial, (2) it is unrealistic, (3) it is an attempt at control, (4) it does not arise from self-respect or kindness to the body, and (5) it leaves no room for the experience of being a complex and growing human being. A remedy for black-and-white thinking is to develop "gray area" thinking, where you let yourself explore the middle ground and the complexity of who you are. You'll also get to open up to kinder ways of understanding yourself and your behaviors. This promotes freedom.

Learning to live in the gray area can initially cause anxiety because we may not feel sure whether we're being "good" or "bad" with our choices and self-care. We've relied on black-and-white thinking for this information before. Yet, with honest reflection, we can see that there were times when black-and-white thinking failed miserably and led to binges. There were times when we broke our own black-and-white rules, just to make ourselves feel bad. And sometimes our black-and-white rules failed to produce the outcome we'd hoped for, and we used that to make ourselves "bad" again.

For example, say we had made the following rule: "Today I won't eat anything before 4 P.M." But we're called in to a special staff meeting where they're serving cookies; we're going to show up hungry, in deprivation mode, and having blood sugar challenges. The cookies are going to look *really* good! Then, once we eat one, the day is ruined. We failed at our plan.

Or say we make this rule: "I'm not going to eat after 6 P.M." Perhaps we feel a little lonely, but we don't know that—we just feel a bit "off," or restless, or bored. Something is gnawing at us and we decide that that was a too-harsh decision. We don't deserve that kind of treatment! We deserve a little bit of ice cream. Then we've shown ourselves to be unaccountable, dishonest, and untrustworthy, to ourselves. (Keep in mind, the rules weren't wise to start with.)

Remembering to first do less harm, then do more good supports us in living in the "gray area" using the following tools:

1. Reduce black-and-white thinking.
2. Reduce good-bad thinking.
3. Acknowledge that sometimes we aren't yet able to do the "best thing," but we are able to do the "better thing."
4. Acknowledge that we cause ourselves harm in ways that we actually can lessen.
5. Be persistent in sticking with the easy ways we care for ourselves.

1. *Reduce black-and-white thinking.* Work on thinking in gray: If you're about to say to yourself, "I will never eat sugar again," as a way to justify a sugar binge, try saying, "I will probably eat sugar again. And I am about to eat it right now. If I make this an all-or-nothing experience, I'm going to really want to overdo this." (You might someday decide you're not going to eat as much sugar, but it will only work when you decide it out of love, not shame.)

2. *Reduce good-bad thinking.* When you don't shame yourself for an "episode" you reduce good-bad thinking. This might feel very awkward at first. And it might seem unbelievable. However, if you don't shame yourself, shame will have less power over you.

When you've had an episode or a slip, your inner dialogue, based in self-empathy and self-forgiveness, might sound like this: "I really regret this. I must have been in pain [or overwhelmed, fearful, lonely . . .]. I didn't know what else to do. My new skills didn't seem like they were going to be as helpful. I feel sad about where I am on my path to recovery. But I know if I damn myself right now, I will give shame more power. And I will be more helpless the next time."

3. *Acknowledge that sometimes we aren't yet able to do the "best thing," but we are able to do the "better thing."* Let's say you aren't able to not eat the "bad food." Eating a "bad food" with complete mindfulness is less harmful to you

than eating in frenzy, numbness, or self-hatred. To eat anything with complete mindfulness means to slow down; explore the flavor, texture, and temperature; notice what it feels like to chew, to swallow, to anticipate the next bite; and for the purposes of "first do less harm, then do more good," it also means to savor the experience fully. Taking away the charge of "good food, bad food" and "good behavior, bad behavior" lets you have the possibility of completely enjoying the food you thought you were going to binge on.

It may also promote the recognition that this food either isn't really that tasty or isn't any more tasty after a reasonable portion. I know binges aren't usually driven by taste, but fully tasting is the "better thing" intervention on a binge and does help us to learn about chosen binge foods. Sometimes we're choosing them for their texture or sound, not just their flavor. (Here I would refer you again to the book *Mindful Eating* by Jan Chozen Bays, mentioned in chapter 4.)

4. *Acknowledge that we cause ourselves harm in ways that we actually can lessen.* If you binge at night, which many people do, and if this bingeing precedes bedtime, which it does for many people, and if staying up late is part of your cycle, you can choose to lessen the harm of one (or all) of these things. In the endeavor to first do less harm, then do more good, choose one of these things to say no to. My recommendation? Say no to the food. Even if you have to stay up past your most helpful bedtime and watch lousy TV, it's not as harmful to you as doing that *and* bingeing. And without the binge, the whole milieu of the activity will begin to change, and will likely become less desirable.

Here is another way you can diminish harm to yourself: get out of bed in the morning as an expression of your self-care. Yoga suggests waking around sunrise in order to establish healthy nighttime and morning routines. (Our cortisol cycles would suggest the same.) For those of you who have well-developed all-or-nothing thinking habits, experiment with getting out of bed "on time" even when you feel like pulling the covers over your head instead.

Or: Make a shift from a toxic substance to a milder substance. For example, reduce caffeine, shift to a sugar that is easier to metabolize, or eat unprocessed food, not Kraft Macaroni & Cheese.

5. *Be persistent in sticking with the easy ways we care for ourselves.* Doing less harm may mean still taking your nutritional supplements even if you don't feel like it. Or sticking with your twenty-minute heart-raising activity — even when you feel like zoning out on the couch — and then letting yourself be a couch potato for a while. (You might need the rest!) It may also mean taking

~~ Interrupting a Binge with Mindfulness

In thinking about my last binge some more, I remembered doing one thing that I don't usually do. I think usually during a binge I enjoy the taste, but in a weird sort of way this is secondary. It becomes more of a task I need to efficiently complete. I have a *strong* internal taskmaster. I think the feeling of fullness is what I am seeking even more than the taste. Then once I feel full, the urge for feeling empty (or purified or cleansed) becomes supreme. This last time, when I was really questioning myself about why am I doing this, I decided to try something different. I challenged myself to shift the focus and to really savor the taste of what I was putting in my mouth. My theory was if I am going to do it, I should at least mindfully do it and it should be enjoyable. During this shift is when I left the "robotic shutdown taskmaster mode." With really paying attention to each bite and the taste and texture I got a surprise. Me, the real awake me, did not really want this at all. After a few bites I didn't want any more. I had had enough and it just didn't taste good anymore. Quite surprising to me really. That is when I stopped. After about ten minutes, I just threw the food away. Not because of something I should or shouldn't do. Because of what I really wanted to do.

— *Kathleen, age 36*

a shower, even when you don't feel like it, or still eating your broccoli even though you binged.

These are fundamentally acts of self-care that move you away from self-harm and toward the ability to consistently do more good. The more you're able to first do less harm, the more likely you are to be able to, and to wholeheartedly want to, do more good! By actively practicing this process, you will greatly reduce black-and-white thinking, get comfortable with gray-zone thinking, and promote recovery, self-forgiveness, and freedom.

THE CYCLES OF RECOVERY AND FREEDOM

Here are two ways to outgrow the cycle of addiction: one is the interventions you can employ immediately anywhere you find yourself on the cycle of disordered eating. The other is the livable pathway out of disordered eating into freedom. The first leads to the second. Let's think of the first as (1) preventions and interventions of your old (disordered) coping mechanisms, and the second as (2) the process of cultivating a life more free of those old (disordered) coping mechanisms.

In much of the literature about addiction and recovery, illustrations representing the "turnout" away from the addictive cycle into recovery are outlined with a mark on the cycle at one place: when a craving arises. The arrow is labeled "new healthy habit" or "new coping mechanism." In the cycle of recovery as I see it, any place on the cycle of addiction is a place for getting out, a place for powerful intervention, not just the place where craving arises. (See the cycle of addiction in fig. 2.1 on p. 17.)

Let's look at how we can use the tool of awareness to intervene in any of these stages in the cycle of addiction and create a turnout onto the path toward recovery.

THE CYCLE OF INTERVENTIONS FOR RECOVERY

- Shame
  Awareness: I am feeling shame.
  To get out: Prevent a shame storm.
  Tools: Ending the isolation (p. 207), returning to belonging (p. 231), awakening self-tenderness (p. 236).
- Use of Survival Strategies
  Awareness: If I start using coping mechanisms, such as black-and-white thinking, eating to the point of pain, and so forth, then I must be feeling anxious or disconnected.
  To get out: Acknowledge to yourself: "I must be anxious. How can I care for myself?"
  Tools: Dashboarding (p. 197), pressure-release-valve breathing (p. 119), fervency yoga poses: structure + heat = transformation (p. 129).
- The Plan
  Awareness: When I see myself making a *plan*, I am on the verge of feeling out of control. Not making a plan will produce a lot of anxiety, yet making the plan will move me to the next stage of the cycle. My plans haven't been sustainable because they aren't realistic.
  To get out: Prevent plan-making.

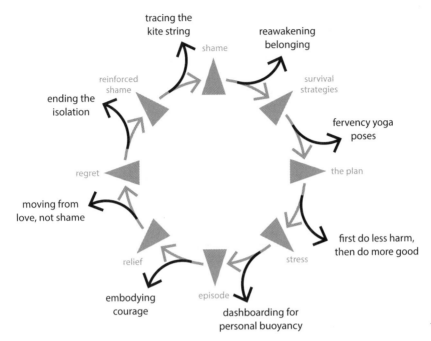

the cycle of interventions
(places to get out)

tracing the
kite string

shame

reawakening
belonging

reinforced
shame

survival
strategies

ending the
isolation

fervency yoga
poses

regret

the plan

moving from
love, not shame

first do less harm,
then do more good

relief

stress

embodying
courage

episode

dashboarding for
personal buoyancy

Figure 8.1

Tools: First do less harm, then do more good (p. 258), sound as mindfulness
   (p. 189), shaking off FFFS (p. 116).

• Stress
   Awareness: I have learned that when I am stressed my body will also be
      stressed and it will have signals. Stress is the red flag before my "episode";
      I can interrupt this if I tend to my body's signals.
   To get out: Recommit to increasing personal buoyancy.
   Tools: Restoring your fuel tank (p. 183), adjusting your physiology (p. 199),
      reconnecting to the source of your vitality (p. 212).

• Episode
   Awareness: If I am already in the episode, I can interrupt it. This is very
      empowering.
   To get out: Claim your courage.
   Tools: Saying *no* to say *yes* (p. 78), embodying courage (p. 172), hot tea mug
      meditation (p. 200).

- Relief

  Awareness: If I got to the relief part of the cycle but I know it is short-lived, it is time to remind myself that in a moment I'll be experiencing terrible regret. Rather than feeling regret that leads to reinforced shame, I need self-forgiveness.

  To get out: Commit to not entertaining shame.

  Tools: Moving from love, not shame (p. 59), nonshaming attitude (p. 110), self-forgiveness (p. 256).

- Regret

  Awareness: If I don't realize I am in the cycle until I am at the regret stage, I can still wake up to what's happening. Regret feels heavy, tragic, despairing. And it makes me feel utterly alone and helpless. Soon I'll be slipping into shame.

  To get out: Prevent regret that spirals to recrimination.

  Tools: Finding faith (p. 147), ending the isolation (p. 207), inflating breath (p. 108), lifeboat of self-empathy (p. 190).

- Reinforced Shame

  Awareness: By the time I get back to this point in the cycle, I may feel hopeless, helpless, and despairing. I know shame can't teach me anything new and won't support me going forward.

  To get out: Get my mind more sane and centered by getting in the GAP, create possibility out of darkness, remember that I am always a learner in recovery (and need not get it perfectly every moment).

  Tools: Tracing the kite string (p. 157), awakening self-tenderness (p. 236), wise humility breathing practices (pp. 124–26).

Freedom

While it's absolutely recovery-saving to know where the "exit routes" are, it is ultimately lifesaving to cultivate the cycle of recovery that frees you from your outdated coping mechanisms. This cycle becomes a spiral of ever-expanding freedom in your life. It is the freedom of being in integrity with yourself, the freedom of knowing you will not self-abandon, shame, shun, or demean. When you have reached this freedom, the tools in this book will be integrated as life skills you use as natural responses to life events. The self-nurturing guidelines won't feel like work. The new discoveries will have become familiar ways of being. Insight becomes action. You will continue to grow and evolve, yet with

the cycle of freedom

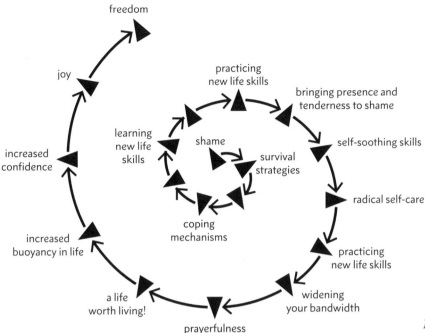

Figure 8.2

tremendous appreciation for the processes of life, and without any sense of urgency or doom. The spiral of this cycle leads to the freedom of living in awe, belonging, wholeness, tenderness, and faith. This spiral toward freedom is characterized by a quiet joy in life, an undercurrent in which you can take refuge. The word *anandamayakosha*, mentioned in the discussion of life vitality in chapter 6, refers to this joy.

To surrender to this possibility requires all of the steps you take on the mountain path of recovery. One of the great tools of yogic surrender is the surrender of who we have been and our compulsion to continually repeat that (to groove our *samskaras*). Through yoga, we also gain the courage to surrender who we think we have to be—meeting the expectations of family or culture, listening to the inner voice of shame, or even pursuing our own agenda—all of which is usually too small to fulfill the spiritual imperative of a 360-degree life. In the process, we even surrender who we might become. At the mountain vista, we recognize how addiction created a too-small life and how recovery is an ever-widening experience of freedom.

- Shame: When shame arises it becomes an opportunity to practice *bringing presence and tenderness to shame.*
- Survival Strategy: Before (or simultaneously) you allow those old coping mechanisms a chance to seduce you with their "pseudo-relief," you employ your *self-soothing skills.*
- The Plan: Once you've employed your self-soothing skills, you'll be geared up to create, employ, and enjoy *radical self-care.*
- Stress: Because you won't be creating a plan that is fundamentally setting you up to fail, you'll find yourself outgrowing your life's previous bandwidth, old patterns, and comfort zones. You'll encounter a new stress instead: the stress of new horizons. Here, you'll respond skillfully by *widening your bandwidth.*
- Relief: As you discover you are acclimating to the new horizons, you will arrive at the heart's expression of *prayerfulness.*
- Increased Confidence and Clarity: As your life becomes more worth living, you'll experience *increased confidence and clarity.*
- Joy: The cycle becomes a spiral expanding outward into *freedom in joy.*

Bringing Presence and Tenderness toward Shame

As we discussed in the previous chapter, one of the remedies for suffering is to reawaken tenderness. In recovery, we will still experience surges of shame. Recovery challenges us to remember how much pain shame has caused and can cause, and to respond very deliberately. First, we become aware of how shame feels in our body: a hot flash, nausea, changes in breathing, or increased tension in muscles. Next, we get present to how shame affects our mind: our mind may become driven (to defend, explain, grasp for understanding, and so on), disoriented, flustered, disturbed, distracted, or dull. Then we become present to how powerfully shame has driven our behavior to get away from pain.

Rather recovery teaches us to turn toward ourselves with tenderness when we're under a shame storm. We may say to ourselves, "This is shame trying to get me. Look how powerful this has been all this time. It's no wonder I've been unable to free myself from this before now." Or we might say, "I know shame cannot now and never has told the truth about me. All this time, I've been under the influence of shame and didn't know it. Today I can get present to how painful this is. I forgive myself for not knowing what to do differently. For right now, I will not let shame win." Ultimately, the ability to talk to yourself this way grows into a great resilience against shame's ability to intrude on your recovery. It also becomes a voice of tenderness toward shame itself, whether it is your own or another's, such as, "Wow, shame has driven so many people to painfully disconnect from themselves. I see now how shame is a cultural web, not just my own. Today, I can be one less person under the spell of shame, for my own benefit and for the benefit of those who may not be able to free themselves right now."

Self-Soothing Skills

Learning the art of healthy self-soothing is one of the greatest gifts of recovery. Because recovery requires us to get comfortable feeling uncomfortable, it will also require us to learn how to get comfortable feeling comforted, how to self-soothe using skillful means. Essentially, self-forgiveness is an act of self-soothing. Yet, as with other aspects of recovery, having a tool that includes body-centered activities builds our ability to directly experience the tool. To only know the tool mentally will not be enough. In a pinch, the mental (cognitive, intellectual) tool can be a terrific reminder. And as we get better at self-soothing, the mental tool can very powerfully tide us over during rough patches.

Just as you were previously able to think of a binge food or food-based coping mechanism and have it bring you immediate relief—for instance, you're in a meeting feeling insecure about your presentation; you have an urge for a cookie; you realize you *will* have that cookie later; you feel less agitated about your presentation—now, thinking about a healthy self-soothing skill can actually bring you a similar immediate relief. In this case, it is the relief of knowing (1) you will not self-abandon, (2) you are becoming a source of security and soothing for yourself, (3) your need for soothing isn't being made bad or wrong, and (4) your need for soothing isn't going to be exponentially postponed. Your consistent response to your valid needs for soothing will greatly deepen your body's ability to trust you.

Here are some of the self-soothing activities my students and I have on our list (note that they all include a sensory-body experience): listening to special music, drinking a quiet cup of tea, petting the cat or dog, curling up with a favorite blanket, sitting by a warm fire, going to a place of beauty, feeling the needles on evergreen trees, dipping hands in a cool clear stream, taking a hot bath, enjoying an early bedtime, using scented body lotion, getting a pedicure or manicure, resting in a hammock, talking on the phone with a trusted friend, connecting with your Attunement Network (as discussed in chapter 6), walking outside in nature, enjoying art or hobby endeavors that stimulate your right brain hemisphere, and gardening.

Radical Self-Care

Radical self-care doesn't imply upsetting others or becoming a "radical" person. The emphasis is on preventing previous thought-strategies from insidiously finding their way into how you care for yourself and promoting a radical commitment to self-care. The commitment I'm referring to here can feel like a radical change of perspective — one in which your recovery is at the center of your commitment rather than constantly compromised by old thought-strategies. Previous thought-strategies may have included self-postponement, "always" putting others first, giving up on your personal commitments to your well-being because it makes someone else uncomfortable, falling into the deprivation-reward mentality, or engaging in black-and-white thinking. Each of these thought-strategies promotes a risk to your recovery. Radical self-care prioritizes your recovery and promotes your body's intelligence, your self-worth, and the preservation of the strides you're making.

RADICAL COMMITMENTS TO SELF-CARE

- *Boundaries:* Limit your exposure to triggers in the form of people, substances, activities, or stimulation (Internet, news, certain conversations).
- *Refuge:* Many meditation traditions recommend that students participate in regular retreats. I call this refuge. In refuge, we become the safe harbor for ourselves. To create refuge, schedule white space (see p. 70) preemptively, well in advance of registering a need for it. Be willing to cancel commitments or reschedule obligations in exchange for a recovery-saving time-out. Create a space in your home or office for this refuge. You may have a place you can sit, lie down, or rest. You may create an altar with art, images, a flower vase, or other objects that remind you of the path you're on.
- *Ferocity:* When boundaries and refuge aren't enough and you're still under the possible threat of previous thought-strategies, it's time for ferocity. Call to mind the fierce protective energy of a mother bear and use it to keep shame at bay during the storm. Use your befriending, homecoming, melt-

ing, or inflating breathing practices from chapter 4, paired with a mantra (a repeated phrase) you create. Some of the mantras that my students have used include:

Stay here in this world [meaning the world of recovery, not shame].
I am moving toward Love [or God, or Freedom, or _____].
This is *not* yours to take! [speaking back to shame]
Only this [I need survive only this moment].
Two toeholds [from chapter 5].
Just for this moment [from chapter 4].
I am saying *no* to say *yes* [from chapter 4].

Widening Your Bandwidth

At this juncture, you will be actively able to open your bandwidth toward your 360-degree life. Our personal bandwidth is akin to our comfort zone with the added consideration of how far we're willing to let that comfort zone stretch. We generate a comfort zone out of our conditioning — familiar, cultural, historical — and our bandwidth reflects to what extent we allow that to be expanded before we feel we need to retract back to our familiar comfort zone. Beyond our bandwidth lies our recovery. Hidden within our comfort zone lie our deeper issues.

In the process of recovery, you will necessarily meet the underlying issues that have been stumbling blocks for you before, but you'll see those hurdles as opportunities to outgrow old limitations and grow into new capacity. And you'll be equipped with the tools to keep moving forward. You will also automatically discover the deeper hungers of the heart that are your life's response to the question "What are you hungry for?" Again, you'll be prepared to handle the excitement and trepidation (remember, they're physiologically similar) that arise in this encounter.

To put this into a visual frame that may help, let's return to our image of the 360-degree life (see p. 5).

A life bandwidth under the siege of disordered eating patterns necessarily becomes smaller. Disordered eating patterns, and all the ways in which we self-medicate, continually narrow our capacity to experience joy, excitement, and contentment in lasting and integrated ways. We may still have peak experiences, yet we don't maintain the "high." We're also continually blocked from dropping down into our ability to be tender toward painful experiences in life, and the greater steadiness, grounding, and poignancy that often comes with those experiences. Poignancy is the tenderheartedness we experience when we realize the vulnerability of humans everywhere to succumb to painful conditioning and a too-small bandwidth. Poignancy also arises when we realize the fleeting nature of life, the preciousness of our journey through all the stages of growth, and the recognition of the courage it takes for any heart to make the climb.

To welcome a painful expression of human conditioning is to close no one aspect of ourselves and no one person or thing out of our heart. It doesn't mean we agree with the way painful expressions manifest in their actions. It means we recognize pain as the seed of these expressions. We might say to ourselves:

- All humans have the seeds of anger, envy, greed, animosity, ill will, and hatred.
- I, too, have these seeds.
- Seeds are expressed in small and large ways, yet they arise from the same ground of human conditioning.
- This has been the case for eons.
- I am not a stranger to this.
- I do not need to shun or reject these seeds of expression.
- As I acknowledge these seeds, I lessen the likelihood of their unskillful expression and increase my capacity to understand human conditioning, my own and others', with compassion.
- I am widening my personal bandwidth and lessening unconscious painful expressions in the world.

Recovery develops our innate ability to be more accepting of ourselves and others as our understanding of what it is to be human becomes more and more empathetic. As stated by the ancient Roman playwright Terence, a former slave: "I am human. Therefore nothing human can be alien to me." This simple statement stands through time because it speaks a fundamental truth. As we are recovering our sense of our whole self, we need no longer be frightened of aspects of ourselves that we find unlikable or "unacceptable." This occurs in the growing certainty we have that, at our core, we will not be shunned, rejected, abandoned, nor banished by ourselves. And that that which we find less likeable in ourselves, or others, is a chance to open ourselves to welcome a painful expression of human conditioning to be understood, not denied. Rainer Maria Rilke said, in his famous passage: "Perhaps all of the dragons in our lives are princesses who are only waiting to see us act, just once, with beauty and courage. Perhaps everything that frightens us is, in its deepest essence, something helpless that wants our love."

Prayerfulness

As we outlive a possible threat to recovery and realize our bandwidth is wider, we experience prayerfulness. Prayerfulness is the combination of re-lief and humility. It is a giving thanks to the grace that carries us through a learning curve. It is not the relief of "whew, we didn't get caught." It is the relief we feel when something compressing our bandwidth has been outlived and our heart expands. Humility is not the same as humiliation. Humiliation seeks to make people smaller, more diminished. Humility allows us to rest in the larger support of the forces of intuition and love that have nudged themselves into our psyche to sustain us in turbulent times. Our humility is how we honor these larger forces. Prayerfulness is us bowing our mind to our heart, bowing our smaller, single life to the larger pulse of life, and offer-ing our recovery to the larger community of those still needing to find their way out.

YOGA INQUIRY

Prayerfulness in Action (PB)

- Join your hands together at your heart in the Anjali mudra (prayer position).
- Consciously feel the qualities of relief, grace, and humility.
- Recognize the larger force of life's intelligence, and the forces of intuition and love that guide you.
- As you bow your head to your heart, lift your prayer-position hands so that your thumbs touch your forehead.
- Give thanks for the grace that has carried you.
- Call to mind the many seen and unseen others who still need to find their way out.
- Offer your strength to them. Offer your sobriety to them. Offer your confi-dence and clarity to them.

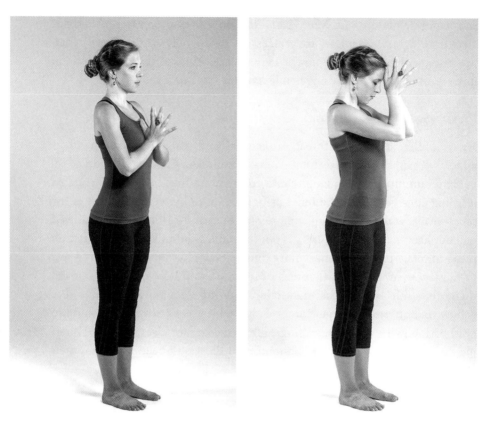

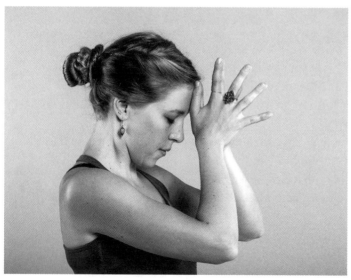

Increased Confidence and Clarity

As you move through these stages you will delight in discovering that your confidence is increasing. You will be less afraid of robotic alien invasions of shame suddenly taking over. Your mind will be steadier. The whims of the scale or other ways you previously measured yourself to find out how you felt on a particular day will no longer have as much power over you. This will also increase your sense of confidence in your recovery.

One of the greatest discoveries, in the realm of your growing confidence, is the realization that your recovery does and will continue to constantly develop in you the deep knowing that you will not let shame win, that you will not self-abandon, and that you are no longer able to justify self-rejection, self-punishment, or self-postponement. You will know more and more deeply that you can trust yourself and the constancy of self-nurturing care and love from which you tend to yourself and all of your needs.

You will also live into a sense of clarity. You will make clearer choices about food, routine, rest, relationships, boundaries, social activities, and so on. You'll find your mind is clearer as your physiology becomes clearer, and that your decisions, while they may be accompanied by trepidation about upsetting someone else, don't leave you with the hangover of angst about your boundaries. This occurs because you become more able to cherish your vitality as the source of how you show up in your life, for both yourself and for others.

When confidence and clarity are restored, you will discover that your capacity in many areas of your life increases, especially your capacity to continue increasing your life skills set, forged through recovery but transferrable to every aspect of living a purposeful, deeply satisfying, and joyful life. Another wonderful discovery: you'll become a lighthouse and a refuge for others. You'll be able to speak about your journey on the mountain path. As you do so, you will further deepen your own confidence in the teachings in this book. (The Attunement Network at my website, www.sarahjoyyoga.com, includes both those in need of persons further along the path of recovery and those who would like to be a lighthouse or refuge for others.)

Freedom in Joy

While our biological imperative has been to survive, our spiritual imperative all along has been to thrive and evolve. From the perspective of our spiritual imperative, we're always on both the journey back home to our innate heart and its capacity for joy, and the journey of wider and wider circles of joy, interconnectedness, and belonging. We flow more toward home, while simultaneously our expression of joy and love flows more outward. Delighted joy, humble joy, radiant joy, poignant joy, and collective joy, as you learned about in chapter 7, are some of the varieties of joy we both experience spontaneously and cultivate deliberately on the journey of recovery. The innate joy of the human heart is that deepest joy that lies beneath all of our suffering and angst, and which supports all of our efforts to rediscover who we are. It is like a magnet of joy pulling us back home to our hearts.

Recovery allows us the freedom to experience this innate joy. Joy is the result of our journey. It is the discovery that this has been our home all along. In the koshas, the center of the human expression is ananda: bliss, radiance, abiding contentment, and joy. Recovery frees us to know this, and to know it free from fear, shame, or questions of worth.

In life before recovery, we may have defined joy as a sort of electric happiness, a jolt of ephemeral experience. Superficial joys are very short-lived. We've all had moments of exquisite joy and peak, fleeting experiences of happiness. Yet two things are in play here that need to be understood: (1) ephemeral joy is dependent on things going our way, or lining up in the external world in such a way as joy is delivered to us; and/or (2) on days when we experienced joy we may experience it as simply good luck. It is as if joy has chosen us in that moment, yet it can as easily be taken away. In this view, joy comes and goes. We're lucky or unlucky.

Recovery through yoga frees us from this mind-set as we are able to directly experience joy from within. This is the joy expressed by ananda. This joy is not coming and going from us. It was not coming and going from us then, nor now. *We* were coming and going from *it*. We were holding ourselves outside the circle of belonging. In recovery, joy is not dependent on external events or circumstances. It is an internal state resulting from the security of knowing you will not be held hostage to shame, of knowing you will not self-abandon, of living in your wider bandwidth, of nurturing your physiological and mental clarity, and from the deep homecoming that you forge in your daily *yes* to that which you know is most true: you deserve this life. The evidence is all around you — most fundamentally in the fact that you exist.

Conclusion

HUNGER, HOPE, AND HEALING

I T SEEMS FITTING THAT I WOULD WRITE THIS conclusion during the last full day of a five-day retreat I'm facilitating for women stepping onto the path of recovery. From the first night, the hunger for relief, understanding, and direction has been palpable. Through these shared hungers, the pain in shared behaviors, and the realization that they are not alone, a sense of safety is established almost immediately for these women. Tonight, I will ask the students to reflect again on three of the things they've been working with daily during their time here: (1) What is something you did well in support of your recovery today? (2) What are the other hungers you've discovered buried beneath your food or body image preoccupations? (3) What are two realistic action-steps you can take in the direction of those other hungers, in the direction of your 360-degree life?

What Is Something You Did Well in Support of Your Recovery Today?

Prior to recovery, you've likely spent more brain space on what you perceive to be your flaws, shortcomings, "not good enoughs," or areas that need self-improvement, and less brain space on acknowledging the courageous steps you are taking. Women are often quick to dismiss a gain that I would acknowledge as significant. And frequently, they're shy in the face of being seen in this courage. Underneath that shyness I see the innocence and earnestness that gets crowded out by self-hatred and the messages from shame. I also see the place in them that is vulnerable to being affirmed. (What if it gets taken away?

What if I can't keep being "good"? What if the expectations go up?) Though we long for affirmation, because it's built into the human organism's desire for assurance about our belonging and safety, we may bury our need for it beneath the pain and the behaviors we use to numb or avoid that pain.

When asked "What did you do well in support of your recovery?" this evening, these were some of the replies:

> "I was able to put my fork down between bites and deliberately taste my food."
> "I obsessed less over what was going to be served for dinner."
> "I felt like hiding out and eating alone. But instead I sat down with two people from the group."
> "I was able to leave food on my plate. Though I was anxious about it afterward (thinking I would get hungry), I didn't. I realized I could try this again."
> "I tried the yoga poses even when I really felt like freezing up."
> "When I felt overwhelmed and judgmental, I focused instead on noticing my feet on the ground and the sounds in the air. It was very freeing. I realized how much energy it takes to be in judgment all the time."

From my perspective, these are all representations of "reviving courage" and "two toeholds in the right direction." Seemingly small things have the power to shift our brain wiring and, as such, our thoughts, attitudes, and actions. In the wind tunnel of shame, there is no step too small to count. It is the strength of the muscles we build in such wind tunnels that makes innate joy surge forth as the wind lessens.

I encourage you to ask the question of yourself on a daily basis: "What is something you did today in support of your recovery?" Write it down as an acknowledgment. Write it in a place you can see it tomorrow (for instance, a note on the bathroom mirror). Affirming what you're doing well, however small you perceive it to be, however great the inclination to dismiss it (habitually or because you struggled on a certain day), is an important step in transforming your relationship to food and your body. You are developing the inner muscle to be a source of encouragement, appreciation, refuge, and confidence for yourself.

What Are the Other Hungers You Discovered Buried beneath Your Food or Body Image Issues?

Early in this book and in each retreat, we ask the questions: "What else might I be hungry for?" "What are the other hungers that food prevents me from knowing about or acting on?" "Outside the 40 degrees of my life that I already know too well (that 40 degrees that represents life under the spell of addiction and shame), for what else might I be longing?"

> *Adventure, spontaneity, playfulness, direction, confidence, ease, contentment, passion, creativity, authenticity, integrity, meaningful friendships, joy, nurturance, honesty, purpose, inner fulfillment, strength, companionship, sovereignty, self-soothing, sweetness, stability, assurance, self-kindness, connection . . .*

I'm always assured that once we start brainstorming this list, the large poster paper on which I write will be too small . . . the words flood the page, energy floods the room. "We do hunger for these things!" I hear in the voice tone of the participants as one calls out a hunger and another adds to it. "This is our birthright!" I see in their body language as one woman affirms another woman's exclamation, "Joy, I hunger for joy!"

The process of giving language to these other hungers opens the life bandwidth for everyone present. Our brains get to hear the language and voice tone of possibility. What lies dormant (tamasic) begins to awaken. Our human conditioning becomes less voluminous as our spiritual imperatives rise in voice, body, and heart.

I invite you to take time to create a list of the possible hungers hidden beneath your food behaviors or body image thoughts. Ask yourself, "For what else might I be hungry today?" If need be, write with your nondominant hand (it can help free your subconscious to contribute). Additionally, you might experiment with asking other people the same question: what are they hungry for in life? Listen for what resonates for you. Consider it a research project on the path to your 360-degree life. Keep your appetite for this question fresh. You can ask this question about hunger(s) at any point along the way of recovery and life at large. It is one of the keys to staying current with your spiritual imperative.

What Are Two Realistic Action-Steps You Can Take in the Direction of Those Other Hungers?

Women often struggle at this point. If the muscle of affirming what you've done well is atrophied and if your curiosity about other hungers has been dormant, you haven't likely exercised this skill on your own behalf. Black-and-white thinking and all-or-nothing thinking will definitely block you from creating success with this. Black-and-white tells you there's one way to move toward a goal and another powerful force dismissing your permission to try. All-or-nothing tells you not to try because you "can't do it 100 percent," or because your life can't create the space or freedom for this, or because it's not okay to risk and fail.

Two of my favorite quotes for recovery are very apt for this juncture:

> I'll tell you how the sun rose — one ribbon at a time.
> — *Emily Dickinson*

> Do not try to do great things. Only do small things with great love.
> — *Mother Teresa*

Here are some examples of action-steps I helped women create tonight:

I HUNGER FOR ADVENTURE:

I could join a hiking group (going once is enough, you need not commit for a year).
I could learn two new or unusual yoga poses.
I could take singing lessons (starting with one is enough, as above).
I could wear colorful clothing one day a week.
I could get a new haircut.

I HUNGER FOR SELF-SOOTHING:

I can take a hot bath.
I can enjoy a quiet cup of tea.
I can create a special place in my home for yoga and meditation.
I can plan a nap into my routine.
I can put a flower or candle on my desk.

If we allow ourselves to arouse curiosity and enthusiasm in the brainstorming list of hungers and we don't follow through, we run the risk of contributing to the tamasic undertow. To create small, achievable action-steps is to build the muscles of self-accountability and faith in yourself as a person on the path of recovery. Remember, however small an action-step may seem, it is unearthing a samskara and reducing its power. Simultaneously you're building new brain pathways. Your outdated conditioning will weaken and your new capacity will continue emerging.

Closing Note

One of the truly amazing (and surprising) joys that arises out of the process of reclaiming your 360-degree life is the retroactive healing that comes with awakening to both your human condition and your spiritual imperative. As you walk through the practices and lessons in this book, affirm the strengths of today's recovery, open your curiosity about the underlying hungers, and take active steps toward those hungers, you will grow exponentially. Your strength, clarity, and ability to love yourself free you from the weight of history, and, with the gratitude that comes with hindsight, you heal the suffering that has caused your pain. What once caused you to shake with apprehension, flush with anger, or collapse into isolation becomes the clear fire of forgiveness toward yourself and others, in both the past and present of your life. What were once profound regrets will become the strength of your sensitivity toward the human condition and your willingness to be available to others in their own vulnerability to suffering. What was once a painful past will become the wisdom and compassion of today.

Appendix

RECOVERY SOUND PANELS

life as a symphony sound panel

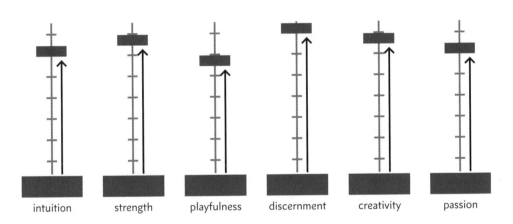

intuition   strength   playfulness   discernment   creativity   passion

some of the instruments in your orchestra

Figure a.1

when addiction skills crowd out other skills

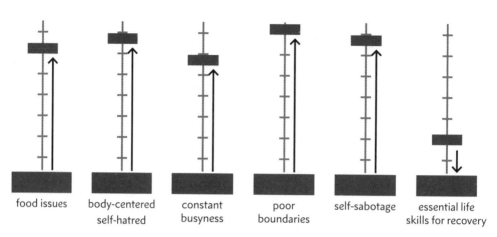

food issues body-centered self-hatred constant busyness poor boundaries self-sabotage essential life skills for recovery

Figure a.2

essential life skills sound panel

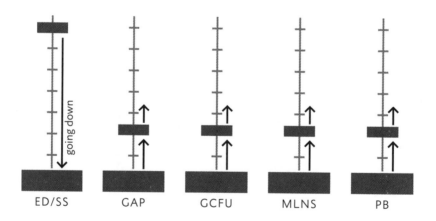

ED/SS GAP GCFU MLNS PB

ED/SS: eating disorder behavior/survival strategies
GAP: getting in the GAP
GCFU: getting comfortable feeling uncomfortable
MLNS: moving from love, not shame
PB: personal buoyancy

Figure a.3

Practices and Short Sequences

Practices

ACTIVE MEDITATIONS

Short Sequences

These are short practices sequenced to provide support for different conditions you may experience or to help as regular home practices to support your recovery.

MOVING FROM LETHARGY TO REVITALIZATION

HARNESSING ANXIOUS ENERGY TOWARD INTEGRATION

Resources

Books

Susan Albers, *50 Ways to Soothe Yourself without Food* (New Harbinger, 2009).

Jan Chozen Bays, *Mindful Eating* (Shambhala, 2009).

Brené Brown, *I Thought It Was Just Me (but It Isn't)* (Gotham, 2007).

Pema Chödrön, *When Things Fall Apart* (Shambhala, 2000).

John Douillard, *The Three Season Diet* (Harmony, 2001).

Cheri Huber, *There Is Nothing Wrong with You* (Keep It Simple Books, 2001).

David Kessler, *The End of Overeating: Taking Control of the Insatiable American Appetite* (Rodale Books, 2009).

Judith Lasater, *Relax and Renew* (Rodmell Press, 2011).

Aimee Liu, ed., *Restoring Our Bodies, Reclaiming Our Lives* (Shambhala, 2011).

Geneen Roth, *Breaking Free from Emotional Eating* (Plume, 1984).

Kathryn J. Zerbe, *The Body Betrayed: A Deeper Understanding of Women, Eating Disorders, and Treatment* (Gurze Books, 1995).

Treatment Centers

Avalon Hills Eating Disorder Programs
Cache Valley, Utah
435-938-6060
800-330-0490
www.avalonhills.org

The Center for Change
Oren, Utah
888-224-8250
www.centerforchange.com

Eating Disorder Center of Portland
Portland, Oregon
888-228-1253
www.montenido.com / edcportland

The Emily Program
Seattle, Washington
Spokane, Washington
Duluth, Minnesota
Minneapolis / St. Paul, Minnesota
888-364-5977
www.emilyprogram.com

Mirasol Treatment Center
Tucson, Arizona
888-520-1700
www.mirasol.net

Rainrock Eating Disorder Treatment
  Center
Eugene, Oregon
310-457-9958
www.rainrock.org

The Renfrew Center
Atlanta, Georgia
Bethesda, Maryland
Baltimore, Maryland
Philadelphia, Pennsylvania
Ridgewood, New Jersey
215-482-5353
www.renfrewcenter.com

Hunger, Hope, and Healing *App*

This portable app gives you immediate access to the tools of recovery, including re-
cordings of breathing exercises, mindfulness tools, and yoga poses. In addition, you can
create your personal 360-degree life chart, track your body dashboard, and create personal action-steps to support your unique journey. Short excerpts from the book keep
you inspired and connected to the teachings and methodologies from *Hunger, Hope,
and Healing*.

Hunger, Hope, and Healing *Online Support*

At www.sarahjoyyoga.com you will find:

• Help creating your personal Attunement Network
• Ayurveda's sleep and daily routine guidelines
• Suggestions for navigating the holidays (or family gatherings, parties, weddings,
  and so on)
• Writing exercises for: Behaviors, Feelings, Needs, and Strategies; Your Two Toe-
  holds Toward Recovery; Creating Your Personal Action Steps
• *Hunger, Hope, and Healing* webinar series

Index

"Wild Geese" (Oliver), 219–20
wise humility, 127, 132
    discipline as, 122–23, 127, 131–32

yoga, xiv
    benefits, 36
    contrasted with other approaches,
        22–23
    documented success, 25–26
    how it helps with recovery, 27
    integrates all aspects of recovery,
        24–25
    is for recovery and for life, 26–29
    nature of, 27–28
    a new lens through which to look,
        35–40
    tripod for recovery, 29–34
    See also specific topics